Starting With Food:

Culinary Approaches to Ottoman History

Edited by
AMY SINGER

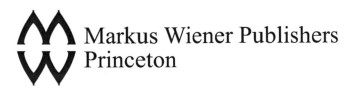

Markus Wiener Publishers
Princeton

Reprinted from Princeton Papers: Interdisciplinary Journal of Middle Eastern Studies, volume XVI, except for the bibliography and index

Cover illustration: "Kaimac Shop in the Tchartchi." From Miss Pardoe, The Beauties of the Bosphorus; illustrations by William H. Bartlett (London: Virtue and Co., [1855?])

For information, write to Markus Wiener Publishers
231 Nassau Street, Princeton, NJ 08542
www.markuswiener.com

Library of Congress Cataloging-in-Publication Data

Starting with food : culinary approaches to Ottoman history /
    guest editor, Amy Singer.
    p. cm.
    ISBN 978-1-55876-513-9 (hardcover : alk. paper)
    ISBN 978-1-55876-514-6 (pbk. : alk. paper)
    1. Diet—Turkey—History—Ottoman Empire, 1288-1918. 2. Food habits—
Turkey—History—Ottoman Empire, 1288-1918. 3. Cookery—Turkey—History—
Ottoman Empire, 1288-1918. 4. Turkey—History—Ottoman Empire, 1288-1918.
I. Singer, Amy.
    TX360.T9S73 2009
    394.1'209561—dc22
                                    2009041425

Contents

List of Figures

"Mr. Turkey Goes to Turkey," Or: How an Eighteenth-Century Dutch Diplomat Lunched at Topkapı Palace

Preface

Food is the basic component of subsistence. Yet at the same time, food is a marker of identity, culture, and class. It can serve to denote relations of power, routine, leisure, and festivity, and document historical change with respect to any or all of these realms. The study of food—consumption, production, distribution, regulation, presentation, preservation, representation—contributes, therefore, to every aspect of historical research. Although this is not a new proposition, it is one that has not been sufficiently developed in the study of Ottoman history. For the most part, the study of foodstuffs has focused on the imperial kitchens and the tables of the wealthy; the large-scale purchase and supply of food to cities, the army on campaign, and the hajj caravans; and the production of food in the context of taxation. However, sufficient evidence exists to expand the scope of investigation considerably, for example: to include the fare of almost every class and each minority or ethnic group in the empire; to examine local regional identities, traditions, and habits as defined by diet; to study foodways and the social organization of meals, together with the symbolic uses and meanings of foods; to consider the texts and uses of law as they pertained to food; and to trace diet and taste from region to region.

Each of the six papers in this volume begins a historical study from the perspective of food, using depictions of food, foodstuffs, recipes, eating habits, meals, utensils, and vessels as the starting point for historical research on the Ottoman Empire. Our collective premise is that these beginnings frame Ottoman history in new and valuable perspectives, whether we are re-examining familiar evidence or stirring new sources into the historian's pot. Indeed, the participants rely on very different kinds of written and material evidence, so that the volume constitutes a series of methodologically distinct but thematically related explorations of how the study of food contributes to the study of the Ottoman Empire in general. The chronological boundaries of our discussion span almost the entire Ottoman era; as a result, the papers address many of the major issues in Ottoman history, all from the perspective of food. Despite the emphasis on the Ottoman Empire in the present collection, we believe that the issues raised by the study of Ottoman history through food contribute as well to comparative, cross-cultural, and interdisciplinary studies.

The papers are organized in roughly chronological order, in order not to impose on the reader any thematic categorization. The themes raised by the articles overlap and intersect, such that it seemed intrusive to subdivide the group. Appropriately, perhaps, it is Nicolas Trépanier's paper "Starting Without Food" which opens the volume. His study of "Fasting and the Early Mawlawī Order" addresses the role of food in writings about the early period of this Sufi order and in so doing discovers aspects of historical change. This is achieved by comparing the intentional abstention from food with the more familiar emphasis on the kitchen and food in discussions of the later Mawlawī (Turkish: Mevlevi) order in the nineteenth and twentieth centuries.

There is a measure of irony in the topic of İklil O. Selçuk's article, "State Meets Society: A Study of *Bozakhāne* Affairs in Bursa," about the sweet, fermented drink called *boza*. This mildly alcoholic beverage apparently held a place of prominence in the commercial and social activities of Ottoman Bursa. Selçuk's study of *boza*, and more specifically the establishments that sold it in fifteenth- and sixteenth-century Bursa, examines taxation, manufacturing, and consumption. Based on several hundred cases involving *boza* that were heard before the chief judge of Bursa, Selçuk also traces the moral and religious critiques of alcohol consumption and the establishments where this took place. It would be interesting in future to compare the newly-investigated case of *boza* with the much-studied history of coffee drinking and coffee-houses in the Ottoman Empire. These latter were also the subject of intense moral and religious debates, as well as suspect for their social functions.

In "Blending In and Separating Out," Rachel Goshgarian uses the portrayal of "Sixteenth-Century Anatolian Armenian Food and Feasts" in Armenian literature to explore the processes of Armenian Christian identity formulation within the larger cultural context of Muslim Anatolia and the war between the Sunni Ottoman and Shi'i Safavid empires. As Goshgarian suggests through the poems she cites, portrayals of food and feasts were drafted into the service of self-definition and confessional boundary-drawing in the charged atmosphere of early modern eastern Anatolia.

Although it may seem anachronistic to construct a discussion of Ottoman public kitchens (*imarets*) under the rubric of a "Michelin Guide," the title of Amy Singer's article is meant to dissociate emphatically the assumed connection between soup kitchens and poor people. Instead, this survey of menus and clients in *imarets* explores the way the distribution of free meals signaled the Ottoman presence throughout the empire, meanwhile defining and reinforcing social and economic hierarchies. Specific dishes, the quantities of food served, and the conditions under which food was consumed each played a part in distinguishing between the clients of an *imaret*.

Tülay Artan explores how the ceremonial and ritual of the imperial hunt and its accompanying feasts stood in for the earlier pageantry and rough living of imperial military campaigns, as well as how they created a similar stage for displaying heroic and martial capacities. This study of "Ahmed I's Hunting Parties" assumes that the narrated descriptions of sixteenth- and seventeenth-century chroniclers were not meant to reproduce a stereotypical image of paradise but rather to relate in concrete detail the conduct of the hunt and the way in which game was tracked and killed, treated, cooked, and consumed. With the chronicle of Mustafa Sâfî, *imam* and confidant of Ahmed I, as a focal text, Artan brings out the contribution of hunting accounts to a nuanced understanding of imperial activities, as well as demonstrating the value of such texts in shaping the image of the sultan.

In the final article of the collection, "'Mister Turkey goes to Turkey,' Or: How an Eighteenth-Century Dutch Diplomat Lunched at Topkapı Palace," Joanita Vroom takes up the way in which meals were served from an entirely different perspective. This study is based on the painter Vanmour's two-dimensional depiction of the event as well as on Vroom's extensive knowledge of material evidence like ceramics, tableware, and food-related utensils. Such evidence, considered together with travelers' accounts and the details of Ottoman and European etiquette, is the basis for tracing the implications of a banquet served by Sultan Ahmed III.

This volume originated in the presentations made at a symposium conducted in Spring 2007 at the Research Center for Anatolian Civilizations of Koç University in Istanbul. The papers were further reworked for a panel at the 2007 Middle East Studies Association Annual Meeting held in Montreal. We would like to acknowledge the contributions of our formal discussants on each of these occasions, Tülay Artan and Cemal Kafadar, respectively, as well as the comments of the audiences and our readers. Our sincere thanks to Markus Wiener for his interest in this volume and to and to Bill Blair, Janet Stern, and Cheryl Fink for the attentive care they have given the manuscript in preparing its publication.

Amy Singer
Tel Aviv University

Starting without Food: Fasting and the Early Mawlawī Order

NICOLAS TRÉPANIER

The work of a historian centers on documenting, analyzing, and interpreting historical phenomena, but it also includes the task of identifying phenomena that previously had escaped scholarly attention. As the present collection of articles abundantly demonstrates, the study of food and food-related activities provides historians not only with a wide and interesting range of topics to study, but also new ways to approach these topics. This article offers a case study showing how an interest in studying food brought to light a hitherto neglected issue, the evolution of Mawlawī practices and identity markers.

The Mawlawī Sufi order finds its roots in the social circles surrounding the mystical poet Mawlana Jalal al-Din Rumi (1207–73), his spiritual associates, and his descendants. Although both this organization's famous originator and its signature ritual (the *samā ʿ*, or whirling dervish ceremony) have made it one of the better-known Sufi orders in the West, scholarly work on its history remains surprisingly narrow in focus. Of course, much has been said and continues to be said about the poetry and outlook of Rumi himself. Yet for all the flowering of literary and theological discussions, comparatively little attention has been paid to the way those who saw themselves as the direct followers of the master received, interpreted, and turned these teachings into rituals over the following half-millennium.

As if bound to classical forms, scholarly accounts of the order itself almost systematically concentrate on a limited list of subjects. At the top of this list is the *samā ʿ* itself, approached either as a religious ritual, as a form of dance, or for the musical tradition that accompanies it. Some studies further discuss (or, more accurately, describe) the various stages through which a Mawlawī disciple had to journey in order to become a member of the order and rise through the hierarchy.[1] However, these Mawlawī rituals are typically presented as traditions independent from any historical context, and one has to read between the lines to realize that the picture given corresponds to the practices of the order in the last decades of its existence.[2] The only aspect of Mawlawī history that is truly cast in a chronological perspective is the succession of its leaders throughout the Ottoman period.[3]

The reasons for such a limited set of subjects in the scholarship on the Mawlawī and for the near-absence of any historicization of its structures and rituals can readily be found in the combination of two factors. The first factor is the nature of the sources. Most of the documentation we have comes to us in the form of theological treatises and poetic works (difficult to approach for one concerned with matters falling outside the explicit domain of religious or intellectual history); hagiographical or biographical accounts of the various leaders of the order throughout its history; and eye-witness accounts of the order in the last few decades before it was legally banned in 1925. The second factor limiting the variety in scholarship is the still too common tendency among historians of the Ottoman Empire to concentrate on the explicit subject of the sources they are using.[4]

We are therefore left with an image of the Mawlawī order's history that is limited to its contour: the greatness of its founding fathers, the uppermost layer of its hierarchy over the centuries, the form of its rituals shortly before it was severed from the social fabric of the budding Turkish Republic. As a general anatomy lesson that would only be skin-deep, little discussion arises about the inner workings of the institution as living organism evolving through history.

But the usefulness of a historical source need not be limited by the topical preferences of its original author, and asking the right questions can elicit answers from unexpected corners. In this article, I will examine a number of sources, especially though not exclusively hagiographies, in order to discuss life within the rank and file of the Mawlawī order. More specifically, I will address the issue of how one particular ritual, fasting, defined the social persona of the order in its early times, despite having left no traces among later generations of Mawlawīs.

Fasting in Late Medieval Anatolian Sources

Any claim that the Mawlawī order entertained a special relationship with fasting has to be examined against the backdrop of the society in which such a relationship developed. The image of fasting in sources from the period allows us, in part, to flesh out such a context, and my first task will consist in providing such a discussion. However, as in any other medieval society, only a tiny proportion of the late medieval Anatolian population is represented among the authors of these sources. Despite this limitation, I will also try to determine which ideas and practices were associated with fasting in the worldviews of the population at large.

The sources consulted as part of this investigation comprise the bulk of the original Persian, Arabic, and Turkish texts produced in the late thirteenth and in the fourteenth centuries in Anatolia.[5] These texts contain a number of depictions of people engaging in fasting. A typical example can be found in the *Maqalat-i Sayyid Harun*, a hagiography describing the foundation of the town Seydişehir (southwestern central Anatolia) in the first quarter of the fourteenth century. The scene depicts a religious master who, in grief, retreats to a cell he ordered to be built into the corner of a mosque: "He would rest his head on a stone and lay on the ground. He would perform the daily prayers with the community, from inside the cell. He spent the rest of his life there. He would eat one iota of food every forty days."[6]

In this anecdote, fasting appears as a way to emphasize the extreme piety of this particular master, a piety that sets him apart from the rest of the population. It is presented along with other elements playing the same rhetorical role, such as using a stone for a pillow and living in physical isolation from the rest of the community. Any one of these elements could be removed from the text without changing the fundamental message of the anecdote. Fasting, in other words, is a device that contributes to creating a particular atmosphere and, therefore, highlights the saintly character of this religious master.

A number of literary devices or motifs, from prayer to the dispensation of charity, play a similar role in these sources, regularly appearing in combination with each other. Just as in the example above, such miniature symbols of piety typically occur in ways that make them ornaments rather than central elements of any particular passage. Removing one of these symbols from the text, in other words, may change the degree of emphasis on the piety of the individual depicted, but it would not affect the character of this piety nor the message conveyed by the passage in which it appears.

This pattern of depiction of fasting is so systematic that I could find but a single case that clearly departs from it. The anecdote occurs in the *Manaqib al-Qudsiyya*, a verse hagiography mostly devoted to Baba Ilyas Khorasani and the revolt he led against the Seljuk authorities in the first half of the thirteenth century. The particular passage discussed here centers on Mukhlis Pasha, the son of Baba Ilyas, after he is captured by an evil ruler who orders that he be put in jail and left hungry for a hundred nights and days. The text specifies that during those hundred nights and days Mukhlis Pasha does not feel any hunger.[7]

In contrast to the pattern I described above, this episode does not refer to fasting in the strictest sense, insofar as it involves imposed rather than voluntary deprivation of food and drink. Furthermore, such "imposed fasting" takes center stage here, and the other narrative elements of the passage (such as the mention of incarceration and of its duration) are subordinated to it. Most important, however, is the mention that the character did not *feel* hunger. The relevance of this latter point will become clearer later on, as we discuss the arguments supporting the positive popular views on fasting. For the time being, I shall simply add the suggestion that this episode, with its "fairy tale" tone, may in fact have been representative of popular epics that were orally transmitted in late medieval Anatolia without reaching us in the particular form they took at the time.

Fasting in the General Population

While most depictions of fasting in the sources involve the great religious masters and saints, it remains relevant to ask whether the general population also engaged in the activity. Of course, the first idea that comes to mind when discussing fasting in a Muslim society is the religious requirement to fast in daytime throughout the month of Ramadan. In this respect, the most striking characteristic of the sources I consulted is the relatively limited number of references they contain to such a ritual, and the emphasis that these few cases put on the *iftār* (fast-breaking evening meal) rather than fasting itself.[8]

A common trait among these references is that they all depict scenes taking place among the political and religious elite. It would of course be unwise to assume that elite behavior, as systematic as it may have been, reflected a corresponding practice in the lower echelons of the social ladder. After all, members of the elite had comparatively easy access to formal, intellectual interpretations of Islam—in other words, an Islam that is closer to the scholarly tradition that prescribes fasting during Ramadan in the first place. Furthermore, it is worth remembering that the beginning and end of the month of Ramadan are determined on the basis of a lunar calendar, shifting approximately ten days every year in relation to the seasons. As a popular religion, Islam was a relative newcomer in late medieval Anatolia, where a largely Christian indigenous population had been organizing its life around a solar calendar until two or three centuries earlier. It would seem reasonable to imagine limitations on the diffusion of a religious festival based on chronological markers that were not only foreign to the Christian population, which may still have formed the majority in the period discussed here, but also at odds with the concerns of the rural segment of the Muslim population, for whom seasons were of far greater importance than the phases of the moon and who had much fewer, if any, opportunities to get in contact with formal Muslim institutions such as mosques or dervish convents.

As a matter of fact, those references to the month of Ramadan I could find tend to appear either as chronological markers or as designations of that month as a moment of heightened piety. However, even among such mentions, few if any offer hints of a popular involvement in fasting during that month. For example, *waqfiyya*s (deeds of pious endowments) from the period often contain prescriptive statements on the use of the endowment's revenues to provide meals to a given (Muslim) religious community, its visitors, and its neighbors. Yet while some of these documents contain special food-related provisions for certain days of the week or certain annual celebrations (for example, buying honey, butter, and flour to make *ḥalwā'* on the two *bayram*s or *'īd*s), those provisions that appear in explicit relation to Ramadan do not require any change in the nature or schedule of meal, despite the fact that this month is arguably the section of the religious calendar most likely to affect food distribution.[9] Absence of evidence is, to be sure, limited ground to assume the corresponding absence of a given phenomenon from reality. Still, this discussion should at least make us wary of facile, undocumented depictions of the period as being marked by a fundamental social divide between by-the-book Christians and by-the-book Muslims.

In any case, I could find only one passage that raised the possibility of fasting *outside* Ramadan by people who were not "religious professionals," namely the peasants of a Cappadocian village. It appears as part of an anecdote from the *Vilayat-nama*, in which the saintly figure Haji Baktash Vali casts a spell on a heap of wheat grain and a heap of lentils. He then turns to the population of the village and says that childless women should pick up one grain, fast for three days (including the night from Thursday to Friday), and put the grain in the mouth of their husband who should not chew it. They will then become pregnant with a boy if they used wheat and with a girl if they used lentil. He further adds that they should make an offering to a saintly figure during the pregnancy.[10]

Such a reference to ordinary people fasting (or, more accurately, being encouraged to fast) is reminiscent of the "atmospheric" role discussed earlier in the case of saints. Just as in the example offered above, fasting here serves to demonstrate piety without playing the central role in the anecdote, nor, in this particular case, in the miraculous ritual. While this reference opens the possibility that people would engage in fasting as an exceptional demonstration of piety for exceptional circumstances, one of its most striking characteristics might indeed be its unique character in the sources consulted. We should therefore not overestimate its representativeness of social practices at large. Another element to keep in mind is that such a recipe for a miracle is directed towards the "civilian" population of a village, rather than to the immediate community of followers of a saint. The importance of this latter point will become obvious in the following pages, as we discuss the place of fasting among the Mawlawīs as a religious order. For the time being, let us simply state that among the general population, fasting was not a widely practiced activity outside and, at least in the countryside, perhaps even during the month of Ramadan.

Justifications for Fasting

Beyond the modalities of fasting depiction and the sheer question of whether fasting is or is not depicted in the sources, it is also important to examine the justifications that these sources ascribe to the characters they depict as fasting. In most cases, such justifications remain implicit, leaving us with the strong impression that the audience was expected to know that fasting was good and to have a good idea of the reasons for such a positive evaluation. Yet here and there, one can find hints of the theoretical grounding that was thus implied. Put together, all of these hints suggest that what made fasting a good thing was that it constituted a form of struggle against the *nafs* or carnal soul. Voluntary deprivation of food and drink, in this perspective, improves spiritual health, purifies the soul, and makes one deserve the rewards of the afterlife.[11] All the narrative depictions of the act of fasting I could find are either hinting at, or compatible with, such a perspective.

Such a presentation of fasting as a weapon against the *nafs*, of course, is by no means exclusive to late mediaeval Anatolia, since it appears in religious discourses throughout most of Islamic history. It is not exclusive to fasting either, condemning as it does all manner of physical pleasures and comforts, starting with plentiful sleep. Yet the depiction of fasting as a form of struggle against the carnal soul also appears, in an unusually explicit fashion, in the book of spiritual advice entitled *Gharib-nama*.[12] That this text was most probably read to, if not *by*, large, popular audiences suggests that, far from being confidential and limited to the intellectual elite, such an understanding of the virtues of fasting was widespread in the population at the time.

In any case, this discussion of the theory and practice of fasting among the general population of late mediaeval Anatolia (i.e., outside of the Mawlawī circles) can be summarized in three points. First, there was a general agreement that fasting was, from a religious point of view, something good. Second, there was also a general agreement that the reason why fasting was a good thing was that it was part of a struggle against worldly desires by exceptional people (i.e., the legendary religious masters) and perhaps, though to a much lesser extent, by ordinary people at exceptional times. And third, there seems to have been little, if any, regular and widespread practice of fasting among the general population, at least outside the month of Ramadan.

Fasting among the Mawlawī

Having established the backdrop of our story, let us now turn to the particular status of fasting in the Mawlawī order. The following analysis is essentially based on the *Manaqib al-'Arifin* and the *Risala-yi Sipahsalar*, two hagiographies of early Mawlawī masters written between the late thirteenth and the mid-fourteenth century.[1] Two main factors justify my choice to concentrate on these two texts, rather than the poetic and theological works of Rumi himself. For one, a certain universalism permeates the personal religious outlook of the latter, whereas a corresponding perspective does not appear to have been as salient among the members of the Mawlawī order. In fact, there even are reasons to believe that Rumi was at least uncomfortable (if not downright opposed) to the idea of a formal, exclusive religious organization being established around him. A reader is of course much less likely to find elements of religious identity setting his followers apart in the works of a man who did not want his followers to be set apart in the first place. Rumi's writings are therefore less relevant material for a study of the Mawlawī order. The second reason to concentrate on these two hagiographies is that the observations and accounts they contain often reveal information that their authors did not care (or even want) to emphasize. Hagiographies, which are by nature subtly yet intensely rhetorical works, take it upon themselves to defend the masters they praise against criticism from their opponents, therefore leaving us with some hints of the nature of such criticism. Rumi's poetic works, on the other hand, are grounded in a long intellectual and literary tradition and use metaphors that very much obscure the particular context of late medieval Anatolia. For example, references to parrots eating sugar appear in his celebrated *Mathnawi*, but rather than representing the patterns of sugar consumption in the context where these verses were composed, they are in fact literary motifs that frequently appear throughout the Persian-language poetic tradition. By contrast, the hagiographies mentioned here contain suggestions that Mawlawīs would inaugurate their fast by ingesting purgatives in order to empty their stomachs;[1] such practical detail is of central importance when discussing the rituals of the early Mawlawīs, yet unlikely to show up in a *Mathnawi* devoted to the celebration of the union with God.

The following table lists all those mentions of fasting that include a reference to duration from both of the aforementioned hagiographies:

TABLE 1

Duration of Mawlawī fasts

Fast duration	Person fasting
1 day	Shams Tabrizi (prescription to his followers).
2–3 days	Fatma Khatun (mother-in-law of Rumi's son Sultan Valad)
3 days	'Arif Çelebi (grandson of Rumi)
3–7 days	Rumi, as a child
5 to 20 days	Shams Tabrizi, in his youth
7 days	Rumi
10 days	Husam al-Din (Rumi's immediate successor)
10 days	Burhan al-Din al-Tirmidi (one of Rumi's spiritual masters)
10 days	Rumi
10–15 days	Burhan al-Din al-Tirmidi
10–15 days	Shams Tabrizi
10– 30 days	Rumi
15 days	'Arif Çelebi
16 days	Rumi
40 days	Rumi
3 months	Shams Tabrizi and Rumi
6 months (two instances)	Shams Tabrizi and Rumi

Though the durations vary considerably, it is relatively easy to find some order in this list. In the shortest case, Rumi's friend and master Shams Tabrizi enjoins his followers, the rank and file of the early order, to engage in a one-day fast, twice a week. Fasts lasting approximately between two and five days involve either the great masters in their youth, or minor figures of the order. Those lasting for a week or two primarily involve the handful of "founding fathers" of the order, characters who tend to be defined by their asceticism. Finally, longer fasts (up to six months) appear in formulations that are strongly reminiscent of the "atmospheric" depictions I identified above in non-Mawlawī sources. For example, three anecdotes telling us about the reunion of Rumi and Shams Tabrizi present these two masters as locking themselves up in a cell for either three or six months, during which time they do not eat anything.[15] Just as in the model I offered earlier, it is another element (the reunion of the two masters) that lies at the center of these three narratives, with fasting playing the part of an "atmospheric" element reminding us of their piety and disdain for worldly considerations.

It is obvious, even from a cursory look at this table, that most of the durations mentioned are far from impressive, at least when compared to the month-long fast of Ramadan. Though the latter does entail significant effort on the part of Muslims who undertake it, the Ramadan fast remains a religious requirement that most healthy adult Muslims are expected to fulfill—and by no means the kind of accomplishment to turn one into a saint. Yet the Mawlawī hagiographies discussed here are rhetorical texts, and the references presented in this table are clearly meant to serve as proof of the special character of masters fasting for as little as a week or less.

In fact, this apparent contradiction is easily resolved if we understand that the Mawlawī fasts were rituals of a different character than Ramadan-style daytime fasts, as they were taking place in a non-stop, day-and-night fashion. As one tries to imagine oneself abstaining from any food or drink without taking a break between sunset and sunrise, a duration of even three days and nights suddenly appears more impressive—and all the more so as one remembers the use of purgatives before the beginning of the fast, as mentioned above.

Comparison with Non-Mawlawī Groups

Extant sources provide us with very little grounds for comparison between fasting among the early Mawlawīs and within other, similar religious organizations. In fact, only the Baktashi order of dervishes provides us with a comparable hagiography, the *Vilayat-nama*, which presents the life and deeds the order's thirteenth-century originator, Haji Baktash Vali, and of his greatest disciples.[16]

Depictions of fasting in the *Vilayat-nama* stand in stark contrast with their counterparts in Mawlawī hagiographies, in part because of the limited number of references—a total of six, some of which allusive at best. These references to fasting are mostly located prior to the pivotal moment of the text, when the central character settles in the village that now bears his name and ties to the later community of Baktashis begin to appear more frequently (through references to specific rituals or geographical locations, for example). Furthermore, almost all of these references concentrate on Haji Baktash Vali rather than his main disciples or the rank and file of his community.[17]

The handful of references to fasting that the *Vilayat-nama* contains show differences not only in quantitative, but also in qualitative terms. For example, the text includes two clearly independent anecdotes that both begin with a wandering dervish asking a village woman for food. In both cases, the woman ends up offering him not only bread, but also oil, and in both cases the formulation leaves no doubt as to the praise these women deserve for offering such relatively luxurious food.[18] These, and a few other anecdotes, suggest that in the Baktashi perspective, occasional luxury on the plate was deemed quite acceptable. Conversely, an anecdote from the *Manaqib al-'Arifin* depicts Rumi as rebuking a group of his followers for having praised the superb meal they were offered by a statesman, telling them that they should not concentrate on such kinds of physical pleasures, let alone brag about them.[19] Such a contrast, I would argue, already suggests that fasting was promoted as a defining element of Mawlawī identity.

But let us return to the table I already discussed, this time updated to include those depictions of fasting from non-Mawlawī sources that mention fasting durations.

TABLE 2

Duration of Mawlawī (*italics*) and non-Mawlawī (**bold**) fasts

Duration	Character	Source[20]
1 day	Shams Tabrizi (prescription to his followers)	. MA 4/70
2–3 days	Fatma Khatun (mother-in-law of Rumi's son Sultan Valad)	. . . . . MA 5/22
3 days	'Arif Çelebi (grandson of Rumi)	MA 8/41
3–7 days	Rumi, as a child	MA 3/2
5 to 20 days	Shams Tabrizi, in his youth	MA 4/24
7 days	Rumi	MA 3/461
10 days	Husam al-Din (Rumi's immediate successor)	. MA 3/541
10 days	Burhan al-Din al-Tirmidi (one of Rumi's spiritual masters)	. . . . MA 2/5
10 days	Rumi	MA 3/403
10–15 days	Burhan al-Din al-Tirmidi	MA 2/19
10–15 days	Shams Tabrizi	MA 3/10
10– 30 days	Rumi	MA 3/339
15 days	'Arif Çelebi	MA 8/34
16 days	Rumi	MA 3/244
40 days	Rumi	MA 3/403
40 days	Spiritual retreat proposed by Haji Baktash Vali	. . . . VN, folio 51a
3 months	Shams Tabrizi and Rumi	MA 4/9
3 months	Spiritual descendant of Sayyid Harun	SH, folio 24b
100 days	Mukhlis Pasha (jailing anecdote discussed above)	. . . . MQ, lines 895–948
6 months . . . . . . *(two instances)*	Shams Tabrizi and Rumi	MA 4/100 and RS p. 128
2 years	Sayyid Harun	SH, folio 8b-9a

This time the contrast is unmistakable, with the shortest non-Mawlawī fast standing at no less than forty days, and the longest reaching two years. Such difference in durations can be explained by a different rhetorical role played by fasting: On the one hand, the hyperbolic character of non-Mawlawī fasts is part of an attempt at setting the saints that perform them apart from the intended audience. Mawlawī hagiographies, on the other hand, were most likely intended to be read by the members of the Mawlawī order, and the more "realistic" lengths of most of the fasts they depict should rather be interpreted as hints that they were to serve as models or examples that the audience could, if not replicate, at least relate to.

The difference between these two ways of depicting fasting can be best explained by offering an analogy with the difference between elite athletes and superheroes. On the one hand, the accomplishments of professional athletes are at once human but push the limits of human abilities, helping them to create a bond with the audience. The sight of professional footballers or Olympic medalists inspires audiences to engage in sports and strive for excellence—even people who do not have the slightest chance of performing at the elite level. On the other hand, superheroes are fundamentally and in essence different from their admirers, and their deeds inspire dreamy thoughts rather than action: Whereas gyms and swimming clubs see a surge in membership during every Olympic year, superhero movies do not seem to encourage vigilante crime-fighting. Likewise, the Mawlawī model of fasting representation (the "elite athletes of fasting") was meant to elicit emulation among the rank and file of the order, whereas the representation of fasting in other sources (the "superheroes of fasting") rather created a distance between the characters depicted and the audience.

The Mawlawī and the Surrounding Society

Looking at the way fasting is justified also affords us an interesting way to contrast the early Mawlawīs and their contemporaries. Just like other narrative sources of the period, Mawlawī hagiographies provide a limited measure of justification in this respect and, just like in other narrative sources of the period, this justification centers on the idea of a struggle against the carnal soul, incarnated in a rejection of the physical urge to eat and drink more than is strictly necessary to survive.

That being said, a closer look at the arguments invoked or implied brings up an important distinction: the Mawlawī argumentative edifice may *center* on the same idea as in other sources, but it is far from limited to it. In fact, both the *Manaqib al-ʿArifin* and the *Risala-yi Sipahsalar* contain a number of independent lines of argumentation, ranging from the example of the Prophet of Islam borrowed from a hadith to the claim of a shaykh that fasting makes his disciples more obedient, and from a reference to the fetidity of feces as proof of the evils of eating to the depiction of the Mongols, under the Hulagu Khan, managing to conquer Baghdad only after fasting for three days.[21] Such a set of argument seems rather eclectic, to say the least, and indeed it is this very eclecticism that provides a hint of the story behind the Mawlawī attachment. The wide range of the arguments used by the authors of Mawlawī hagiographies seems indeed very much like the outcome of a rationalizing process through which a group of people sought any possible argument in order to justify a practice that had already been adopted. In other words, it appears that the Mawlawī gave fasting a central role as a ritual and as an element of identity long before they began engaging in intellectual deliberations on its subject.

This set of arguments also suggests that Mawlawī authors felt fasting needed to be justified in the first place. As was pointed out on several occasions already, hagiographies are rhetorical texts. While their authors tend to shy away from mentioning the accusations that some opponents may have leveled against their revered masters, they also see it as their duty to defend these same masters against what they considered to be libel. This seems to be precisely the process taking place here: If the authors of the *Manaqib al-ʿArifin* and the *Risala-yi Sipahsalar* were seeking any possible form of argumentative support for fasting, it is because the status of fasting among the Mawlawī was the object of contestation from outside the order.

Given my earlier discussion of the pious image that fasting seems to have enjoyed in the society at large at the time, such a contestation may seem surprising. The root of the problem may in fact not have been the validity of fasting as a religious ideal *per se*, but rather the social associations carried by extreme fasting, witnessed first-hand. At least two of Rumi's masters, Shams Tabrizi and Burhan al-Din Tirmidi, appear to have been associated with the movement generally known as Qalandariyya in their early years. Since the Qalandariyya is mostly known through heresiologies denouncing it, this movement's theological groundings remain difficult to ascertain. Still, it seems clear that social renunciation (deliberate efforts to be rejected by mainstream society) and extreme asceticism were among the most visible attributes of Qalandar dervishes,[22] making them the most visible practitioners of extreme fasting in late medieval Anatolia. Given the high social status of Rumi and of his own family (well-regarded religious scholars and regular visitors at Seljuk palaces since long before any hint of fasting or whirling entered the picture), such an association with a marginal movement promoting the destruction of every rule of etiquette, every physical pleasure, and every luxury had to appear rather shocking to the members of the surrounding high society.[23]

Putting the Mawlāwīs Back in History

The origins of the "Mawlawī attitude to fasting" discussed in this article can probably be found in the meeting between Rumi and Shams Tabrizi, which took place ca. 1244. The same outlook is also pervasive in the *Manaqib al-'Arifin*, whose second redaction (the only one extant) dates from ca. 1353. It therefore seems clear that, within the circle of Rumi's immediate followers and descendants, fasting held a central place for a century at least, from the middle of the thirteenth to the middle of the fourteenth century.

As I pointed out at the beginning of this article, the only substantial studies we have of Mawlawī rituals describe them as they existed in the nineteenth and especially early twentieth centuries. In these depictions, fasting is totally absent as a practice, let alone as a symbol of social identity for the order. In fact, the use that later Mawlawī made of the word *chilla* allows us to go even further in dissociating the later incarnation of the Mawlawī order from the practice of fasting. Whereas most other Sufi brotherhoods typically use this word to designate a forty-day physical retreat involving at least some degree of voluntary food deprivation,[24] the later Mawlawī context gives it a unique meaning, designating a 1001-day period during which a new disciple performs menial tasks in service of the other members of the order, without engaging in fasting.[25]

Such a contrast between early and late Mawlawī practices is far from unique. For example, Gölpınarlı notes a number of cooking-related titles which were given to members of the order in the early twentieth century, at a time when he himself was a member, and notes that these titles were associated with both specific kitchen functions and particular hierarchical statuses.[26] Such a ritualized attribution of food-preparation roles appears totally absent from the description of daily activities in the first century of the organization's life. In fact, one anecdote depicts the attribution of cooking duties to particular dervishes by sheer virtue of these individuals' particular talents and professional backgrounds, suggesting that the hierarchy in kitchen responsibilities that we see in the later order was absent in its earlier generations.[27]

Of course, the notion that rituals were much more detailed and deeply engrained in the routine of nineteenth- and twentieth-century Mawlawīs than they had been for their predecessors six hundred years earlier is hardly surprising. Yet it does entail a historical process of change, a process whose very existence remains unacknowledged by most of the scholarly literature on the history of the order.

The presence of an association between the early Mawlawī order and the practice of fasting thus demonstrates that the study of food, and of the human practices that surround it, can offer what a historian most hopes for: New historical questions and new lines of inquiry that can challenge facile, undocumented conclusions. In the Mawlawī case, after all, how could the order, organized around the kitchen in its later incarnation, have remained unchanging through its "middle centuries" when it started without food?

Notes

1. See for example Abdülbâki Gölpınarlı's seminal study of the order, *Mevlâ-nâ'dan sonra Mevlevîlik*, 2nd ed. (İstanbul: İkilâp Kitabevi, 1983), here pp. 367–408, which was first published in 1953 and partially based on its author's own experiences as a member of the order; see also Shams Friedlander, *The Whirling Dervishes* (Albany: SUNY Press, 1992), pp. 87–93 and 107–10.

2. One might be tempted to characterize as efforts to historicize the *samā'* the attempts that some authors have made to determine the exact moment when the practice was "set" (therefore entering the comforting realm of the "time-less"). For example, Franklin Lewis in his monumental summary of the current scholarship on Rumi and the Mawlawī (*Rumi Past and Present, East and West: The Life, Teachings and Poetry of Jalâl al-Din Rumi* [Oxford:

Oneworld, 2000], p. 461), notes that: "Sultan Valad may have given structure to the Mevlevi order, but not until the time of his grandson, Pir 'Adel Chelebi (d. 1460), did the orders' [sic] rituals assume their basic shape. Since then, however, the only significant change we know of in Mevlevi praxis occurred during the reign of Selim III (1789–1807), which mostly affected the circumstances, locale and frequency of the performance of the *samā* '." Such a presentation of the chronology may be an accurate reflection of the historical data available, but also implicitly disregards any gradual change in rituals that, as the present article seeks to demonstrate, must have happened over the centuries.

3. See for example Gölpınarlı, *Mevlânâ'dan sonra*, pp. 151–81.

4. The most laudable exception to the lack of diversity among the studies of the order is an article by Suraiya Faroqhi ("Agricultural Crisis and the Art of Flute-Playing: The Worldly Affairs of the Mevlevî Dervishes (1595–1652)," *Turcica* 20 [1988]: pp. 43–70), which examines the financial dealings of a number of Mawlawī convents in Anatolia from the late sixteenth to the mid-seventeenth century. The article, like so many others by the same author, is masterfully documented and has the merit of exploring a category of sources otherwise ignored in studies of the Mawlawī organization. However, it remains subject to the second limitation mentioned here, insofar as it is for a discussion of the accounting and fiscal dealings of the order that it uses accounting and fiscal documents.

5. 'Abd al-Karim b. Shaykh Musa, *Maqalat-i Sayyid Harun* (edited by Cemâl Kurnâz as *Makâlât-ı Seyyid Hârûn: Tenkitli Basım* [Ankara: Türk Tarih Kurumu Basımevi, 1991]); Ahmedi, *Iskandar-nama* (edited and translated by Kemal Sılay in "Aḥmedî's history of the Ottoman dynasty," *Journal of Turkish Studies* vol. 16 [1992]: pp. 129–200); Aqsarayi, *Musamarat al-Akhbar* (edited by Osman Turan as *Musamirat al-Akhbar va Musayirat al-Akhyar* [Ankara: Anjuman Tārīkh Turk, 1943/4]); Astarabadi, *Bazm u Razm* (edited by Fuat Köprülü as *Bazm va Razm* [İstanbul: Avkâf Maṭba'ası, 1928]); 'Ashiq Pasha, *Gharib-nama* (edited by Kemal Yavuz as *Garib-nâme: Tıpkıbasım, Karşılaştırmalı Metin ve Aktarma* [İstanbul: Türk Dil Kurumu, 2000]); 'Ashiq Pashazada, *Tavarikh-i Al-i Osman* (edited by Çiftçioğlu Nihat Atsız as "Tevârîh-i Âl-i Osman" in his *Osmanlı Tarihleri* [İstanbul: Türkiye Yayınevi, 1949], pp. 77–319); Elvan Çelebi, *Manaqib al-Qudsiyya fi Manasib al-Unsiyya* (edited by İsmail Erünsal and Ahmet Yaşar Ocak as *Menâkıbu'l-Kudsiyye fî Menâsıbi'l-Ünsiyye: Baba İlyas-ı Horasânî ve Sülâlesinin Menkabevî Tarihi* [Ankara: Türk Tarih Kurumu Basımevi, 1995]; also edited by Mertol Tulum as *Tarihî Metin Çalışmalarında Usul: Menâkıbu'l-Kudsiyye üzerinde bir Deneme* [İstanbul: Deniz Kitabevi, 2000]); Enveri, *Dustur-nama* (edited and translated to French by Irène Mélikoff as *Le Destan d'Umur Pacha*

[Paris: Presses Universitaires de France, 1954]); Gülşehri, *Karamat-i Akhi Avran* (edited by Franz Taeschner as *Gülschehrîs Mesnevi auf Achi Evran, den Heiligen von Kirschehir und Patron der türkischen Zünfte* [Wiesbaden: Franz Steiner Verlag, 1955]); Ibn Battuta, *Rihla* (edited and translated by C. Defrémery and B. R. Sanguinetti as *Voyages d'Ibn Batoutah*, 4 vols. [Paris: Société Asiatique, 1874–79]); *Qabus-nama* (sample of five old Anatolian Turkish translations edited by Eleazar Birnbaum in *The Book of Advice by King Kay Kâ'us ibn Iskander: The Earliest Old Ottoman Turkish Version of his Ḳâbûsnâme*, Sources of Oriental Languages and Literatures 6 [Duxbury, MA: Şinasi Tekin and Gönül Alpay Tekin, 1981], pp. 16–25); al-'Umari, *Masalik al-Absar fi Mamalik al-Amsar* (edited by Ahmad 'Abd al-Qadir al-Shadhali as *Masalik al-Absar fi Mamalik al-Amsar* [Abu Dhabi: al-Majma' al-Thafâqî, 2003]); and *Vilayat-nama-yi Haji Baktash Veli* (edited by Abdül-bâkî Gölpınarlı with a MS. facsimile as *Vilâyet-nâme: Manâkıb-ı Hünkâr Hacı Bektâş-ı Veli*, 2nd edition [İstanbul: İnkılâp, 1995]).

6. "Mescidün köşelerine çilehaneler yapün didi. Yapdılar. Bir zamân geçdi. Dedigi Sultan âhirete gitdi diyü istima' olındı. Sultan gâyet bi-huzur olup gayb namâzını kıldılar. Andan sonra 'cuma mescidi'nün içinde çilehaneden çıkmadı. Taş yasdandı ve toprak döşendi. Namâzı cemâ'atle çilede qılurdı. Bâkî ömrını anda geçürdi. Kırk günde bir zerre mıkdârı ta'âm yirdi." (*Maqalat-i Sayyid Harun*, p. 22a).

7. Elvan Çelebi, *Manaqib al-Qudsiyya*, lines 894–948 (both editions use the same line numbering system).

8. *Ifṭār* is the term commonly used to refer to the fast-breaking dinner during Ramadan. It is true that it sometimes does occur as part of the Persian compound verb "*ifṭār kardan*" with the meaning of "to start eating" or "to eat," without implying any more religious fasting than does the English word "breakfast"; on some occasions, the formulation leaves no doubt that it should clearly be dissociated from the fast of Ramadan (see for example *Vilayat-nama*, fol. 156a—all references to this text, hereafter cited as *Vilayat-nama*, are to the appended MS facsimile, which is different from that appearing in Gölpınarlı's first edition). In other cases, however, the word *ifṭār* does refer to meals explicitly taking place during that month, and it is reasonable to interpret such occurrences as hints that at least some mediaeval Anatolian Muslims fulfilled the duty of daytime fast in Ramadan (see for example *Bazm u Razm*, p. 169).

9. See, for example, the *waqfiyya* from Konya dated 765/1363–64 (Vakıflar Genel Müdürlüğü (hereafter VGM), Ankara: Defter 596, Sayfa 151, Sıra 134,), which provides a special budget for Qur'anic recitations during the month of Ramadan, and a *waqfiyya* from Tokat, also dated 765/1363–64 (VGM: D. 611, Sa. 93, Sı. 79), which provides for candles to be used during the same month.

It would at first glance seem logical to assume that the latter case entails a change in habits congruent with the daytime fast of Ramadan (namely the use of candle for those staying awake later than usual after sunset). However, one should also note that the provision demands that candles be lighted not only during the nights of Ramadan, but also on a number of other days, including every Friday (which excludes the possibility of a systematic association with fasting). This provision closely parallels the prescription, appearing in a Niksâr *waqfiyya* dated 723 AH/1323 (VGM, D. 581/2, Sa. 198, Sı. 300), to light candles on a limited list of festive days that fall both during and outside of Ramadan, but without any mention of the latter or fasting.

10. *Vilayat-nama*, fol. 61a.

11. In the example of Mukhlis Pasha discussed above, the fact that food and drink deprivation was imposed by an outside figure (the evil ruler) rather than being a self-imposed exercise in asceticism indeed suggests a slightly different theoretical grounding, therefore putting the example in a separate category. As much as we are expected to admire the physical deed of Mukhlis Pasha, in other words, the text's specification that he *did not feel* hunger suggests that this was a physical rather than spiritual accomplishment.

12. The *Gharib-nama* seems to have been the first original work written in Turkish in Anatolia, and its author explicitly claims that he chose this language, rather than Persian (popular among the political and literary elite) or Arabic (the religious language *par excellence* among Muslims, then as always), precisely because he wanted a broader reach into the general population, among whom the Turkish language was more common.

13. This, among other things, makes them the best sources we have on the life of Rumi, as well as the likes of his friend and master Shams Tabrizi and his son and successor Sultan Valad. Shams al-Din Ahmad Aflaki, *Manaqib al-'Arifin*, ed. Tahsin Yazıcı, 2 vols. (Ankara: Châpkhânah-i Anjuman-i Ta'rîkh-i Turk, 1961); and Faridun b. Ahmad Sipahsalar, *Risala*, edited by Sa'id Nafisi as *Risala-yi Faridun b. Ahmad Sipahsalar dar Ahval-i Mavlana Jalal al-Din Mavlavi* (Tehran: Kitâbkhâna ve Châpkhâna-yi Iqbâl, 1320/1941-2).

Although *Risala-yi Sipahsalar*, which shares a number of anecdotes with *Manaqib al-'Arifin* (generally showing at least minor changes in formulation), is conventionally said to originate from the turn of the fourteenth century, we do not have clear date for its completion. The scholarly convention claiming that *Risala* not only predates but also served as a source for *Manaqib al-'Arifin* deserves to be addressed in a more critical fashion. For the purposes of this article, however, I have assumed a near-contemporary character for the two texts since, in any case, none of the arguments or conclusions presented here would be significantly different if they were based exclusively on the reliably dated *Manaqib al-'Arifin*.

14. *Manaqib al-'Arifin*, par. 3/40, and *Risala-yi Sipahsalar*, p. 81.

15. *Manaqib al-'Arifin*, par. 4/9 and 4/100; *Risala-yi Sipahsalar*, p. 128.

16. There are of course a number of key differences between the two orders, the Mawlawī showing stronger ties with the urban craftsmen and elite classes, while the Baktashi order seems to have arisen primarily in a peasant context. Such contrast is obvious, among other signs, from the languages chosen for the hagiographies discussed here (Persian for the *Manaqib al-'Arifin* and *Risala-yi Sipahsalar*, and Turkish for the *Vilayat-nama* of Haji Baktash Vali). One should also note that lengthy passages from the Baktashi source clearly were borrowed from other, now lost hagiographical traditions. Of course, this does not prevent them from reflecting the ideology of those Baktashis who are responsible for such imports.

17. The most significant exception is of course the prescription of fasting as a preparation for a miracle, as I mentioned earlier, although one should remember that it involves the peasants of a nearby village rather than the immediate members of Haji Baktash's community: *Vilayat-nama*, fols. 5b, 8a, 23a, 37a–b, 50b–51a, 61a.

18. *Vilayat-nama*, fols. 46b and 49a.

19. *Manaqib al-'Arifin,* par. 3/438.

20. MA: *Manaqib al-'Arifin*; MQ: *Manaqib al-Qudsiyya*; RS: *Risala-yi Sipahsalar*; SH: *Maqalat-i Sayyid Harun;* VN: *Vilayat-nama*.

21. Respectively *Manaqib al-'Arifin,* par. 3/487, and *Risala-yi Sipahsalar*, p. 65; *Manaqib al-'Arifin,* par. 4/79 for the second; *Manaqib al-'Arifin,* par. 3/481 for the third; and *Manaqib al-'Arifin,* par. 3/112 for the fourth. The most extreme case of eclectic argumentation, however, occurs in a discussion (in Arabic, and probably excerpted from a theological treatise which I have not been able to identify) in which Rumi himself gives a list of categories of people (physicians, philosophers, kings, etc.) who all agree on "hunger and little food" (*al-ju' wa qillat al-akl*) as the best practice for themselves, each group of people suggesting a different reason to fast, from an increased concentration to a purification from illness (*Manaqib al-'Arifin,* par. 3/518).

22. The most exhaustive study of the Qalandariyya is Ahmet Karamustafa, *God's Unruly Friends: Dervish Groups in the Islamic Later Middle Period, 1200–1550* (Salt Lake City: University of Utah Press, 1994).

23. The social status of the Qalandariyya seems to have had much in common with that of the twentieth-century hippie movement. Its likely association with Rumi's followers, resulting in tensions that made the authors of the Mawlawī hagiographies so eager to defend fasting, can therefore be likened to the association that the use of LSD created between the hippie movement and Har-

vard professor Timothy Leary, ultimately resulting in the latter's dismissal
from the Harvard faculty.

24. It seems to have been the case among the early Baktashis. See for example
Vilayat-nama, fols. 37a–b and 50b–51a.

25. Gölpınarlı, *Mevlânâ'dan Sonra*, pp. 391–96.

26. Gölpınarlı, *Mevlânâ'dan Sonra*, pp. 396–8.

27. *Manaqib al-'Arifin,* par. 1/21 and 8/85.

State Meets Society:
A Study of *Bozakhāne*
Affairs in Bursa*

İKLİL O. SELÇUK

The manager of the tax-sources of the *bozakhānes* (in Bursa),
Seydi Ahmed b. Resul said the following at the *qadi* court: I took
from İlyas b. Abdullah, the holder of Kanber Bozakhāne, completely and without remainder, the *bozakhāne* down-payment and
the taxes charged toward contractual expenses from the first day
of the *rebiyy'ül-evvel* until the end of *rebiyy'ül-ākhir* in the year
896 Hijrī. The aforementioned *bozakhāne* holder confirmed. The
witnesses: Mustafa b. Mehmed; Mevlana Eyüb; and the scribe of
these letters; and Mevlana Sinan El-Din.[1]

This is one of several hundreds of cases among fifteenth-century Bursa
qadi court records on *bozakhānes*, commercial establishments where a
sweet and fermented drink called *boza* was sold.[2] This particular court
record reveals that by 1491, *bozakhāne* management in Bursa was a tax-
generating activity overseen by officials and, as such, came under the fiscal
supervision of the central government. This paper looks into court cases
from Ottoman Bursa, aiming to highlight various aspects of *bozakhāne*

* I am grateful to Engin D. Akarlı, Özer Ergenç, Cemal Kafadar, Amy Singer, and Nicolas
Trépanier for their comments and generous help with the preparation of this paper.

affairs including the popularity of *boza*, the lucrative nature of the business, state ownership of *bozakhāne* buildings, the heterogeneous identities of the patrons, and moral and religious concerns related to the consumption of this fermented drink in an Islamic society. More specifically, I argue that fifteenth- and sixteenth-century Bursa *bozakhānes* seem to have been among the most popular public places, hosting people of various backgrounds, until the coffeehouses' unprecedented rise in the seventeenth century eclipsed them.

Ottoman court records, allowing us an empirical analysis of the fiscal and administrative dynamics of *boza* affairs in Bursa, indicate that the sources of conflict in *bozakhāne* administration included the production activity itself, the choice of supervisors and tenants, the rental periods, the conditions of rent renewal, the oversight of the alcohol content of *boza*, and the regulation of *bozakhāne* patrons.

Court Records on Bursa *Bozakhānes*
in the Late Fifteenth Century

Where were Bursa *bozakhānes* located? Who were the inhabitants of the districts where *bozakhanes* were established? Were these neighborhoods also significant commercial areas? Did the location of *bozakhānes* affect the rent charged for each? Six *bozakhānes* are found in Bursa court records from 1482.[3] The daily rent they paid to the owner of the work premises, namely the Ottoman state, varied between fifteen and eighty-five *akçes*. Two additional *bozakhānes* joined them in 1485.[4] There are references to seven additional *bozakhānes* in the records of the succeeding decades. In total, Bursa court records of the late fifteenth and the sixteenth centuries mention fifteen different *bozakhānes*.[5]

Following the conquest, the initial Ottoman settlement in Bursa in the citadel (*hisar*) took place rather rapidly. The previous inhabitants of the citadel, the non-Muslims, had to leave this area, and the majority of the churches within the citadel were converted to mosques and *medreses* (schools of religious education).[6] During the early settlement period, these local non-Muslims of Bursa moved to the western and northeastern edges of the citadel.[7] It is likely that the clientele of the *bozakhānes* in these neighborhoods included the local non-Muslim inhabitants of Bursa. Who else frequented these *bozakhāne*s probably depended on the nature of the neighborhood, that is, whether it was in a commercial district or not. With this point in mind, let us now take a closer look at the locations of Bursa's *bozakhāne*s:

Figure 1 shows the historical development of Bursa from Orhan Gazi's time (r. 1324–60) until the end of Mehmed II's reign (1451–81). Figure 2 shows the locations of Bursa's neighborhoods accompanied by a list of the neighborhood names (Table 1). Figure 3 locates some neighborhoods with *bozakhāne*s. Figure 4 shows the commercial centers and significant public buildings.[8]

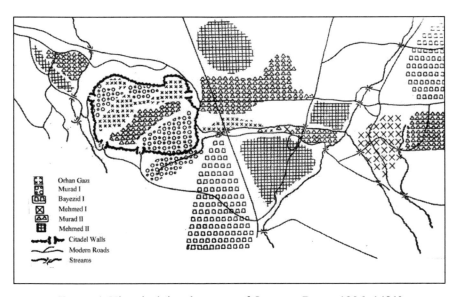

Figure 1. Historical development of Ottoman Bursa, 1326–1481[9]

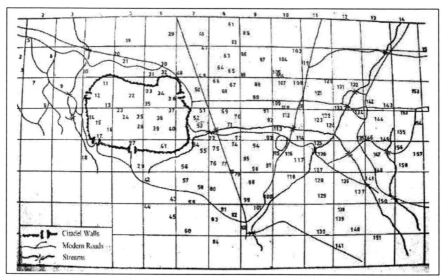

Figure 2. Locations of the neighborhoods of Bursa[10]

TABLE 1

Neighborhoods of Bursa according to divisions on Figure [11]

1	2	3	4
1. Hamza Bey	5. Beşikçiler	9. Kayabaşı	10. Yahşi Bey
2. Bahadır Ağa	6. Muradiye		11. İmāret-i İsa Bey
3. Elvan Bey	7. Azeb Bey		12. İsa Bey el-Fenari
4. Demirkapı	8. Kocanaib		13. Helvacı-oğlu
			14. Alaaddin Bey
			15. Filboz
			16. Tahta Mescid
			17. Zindan Kapısı
			18. Alaca Hırka

5	6	7	8
19. Istabl-i Bayezid	29. Ahmed Paşa	46. Hacı Yakub	61. Kiremitçizade
20. Altıparmak	30. Şehabeddin Paşa	47. Doğan Bey	62. Simitçi

21. Veled-i Kazzaz	31. Kuruçeşme	48. Veled-i Sarayi	63. Veled-i Mizan
22. Tefsirhan	32. Çatalfırın	49. Şehreküsdü	64. Narlı
23. Nakkaş Ali	33. Manastır	50. Hacı İlyas	65. Zağfiranlık
24. Şeyh Paşa	34. Kal'a Camii	51. Sağırnıc Sungur	66. Mantıcı
25. Satı Fakih	35. Orta Bazar	52. Balıkbazarı	67. Reyhan Paşa
26. Kal'a-ı Umur Bey	36. Darbhane	53. Bilecik	68. Veled-i Enbiya
27. Molla Gürani	37. Şahin Lala	54. Debbağhane	69. Bedesten
28. Pınarbaşı	38. Veled-i Yanic	55. Hacı Sevinç	70. Uzunçarşı
	39. Çerağ Bey	56. Veled-i Veziri	71. Cami'-i Kebir
	40. Kavaklı	57. Konurzade	72. Mecnun Dede
	41. Yerkapı	58. Araplar	73. Orhan
	42. İzeddin	59. Teke Mescid	74. Şeker Hace
	43. Hacı İvaz Paşa	60. Uçkuz	75. Tahtakale
	44. Seyyid Nasır		76. Duhter-i Şeref
	45. Kızılcabayır		77. Ebu Şahne
			78. Arab Mehmed
			79. Veled-i Habib
			80. Ali Paşa
			81. Kademleri
			82. Düsturhan
			83. Şeyh Hamid
			84. Molla Fenari

9	10	11	12
85. Hacı Menteş	103. Kassab Hüseyin	119. Timurtaş	131. Kanberler
86. Suzen-i Kőfn	104. Hace Yunus	120. Kız Yakub	132. Atbazarı
87. Daye Hatun	105. Acem Reis	121. Ebu Ishak	133. Ahmed-i Dai
88. Yeni Bezzaz	106. Kepezler	122. Kőseler	134. Meydancık
89. Elmalık	107. Abdal Mehmed	123. Kaygan	135. Yeşil
90. Yiğid-i Cedid	108. Hasan Paşa	124. Kirişçi Kızı	136. İshak Şah
91. Tuzpazarı	109. Hayreddin Paşa	125. Selçuk Hatun	137. Hacı İskender
92. Simkeş	110. Karakedi	126. Kurdoğlu	138. Umur Bey
93. Kara Şeyh	111. Yiğid-i Kőhne	127. Sedbaşı	139. Veled-i Bevvab
94. Veled-i Nalband	112. Şerafeddin Paşa	128. Karaağaç	140. Çoban Bey
95. Veled-i Hariri	113. Sarı Abdullah	129. Hace Mehmed Karamani	141. Eşrefiler

96. Akbıyık	114. Hace Tayyib	130. Temenna
97. İbrahim Paşa	115. Hacılar	
98. Veli Şemseddin	116. Alaca Mescid	
99. Başçı İbrahim	117. Hoşkadem	
100. Sivasiler	118. Hoca Alizade	
101. Çardak		
102. Maksem		

13	**14**	**15**
142. Tatarlar	152. Mücellidi	159. Yıldırım
143. İncirli	153. Veled-i Bezzaz	160. Çukur Mescid
144. Hacı Sevindik	154. Emir Sultan	161. Hacı Seyfeddin
145. Bayezid Paşa	155. Fazlullah Paşa	162. Zeyniler
146. Sultan Mehmed	156. Taşgu	163. Pir Emir
147. Şeyh Şibli	157. İnceğizler	
148. Baba Zakir	158. Karamazak	
149. Mesud Mekramavi		
150. Namazgah		
151. Molla Arab		

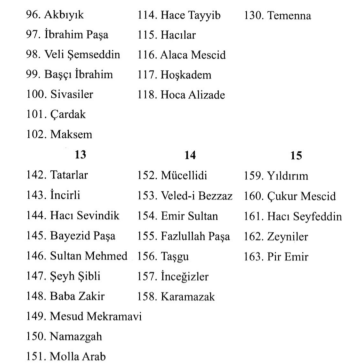

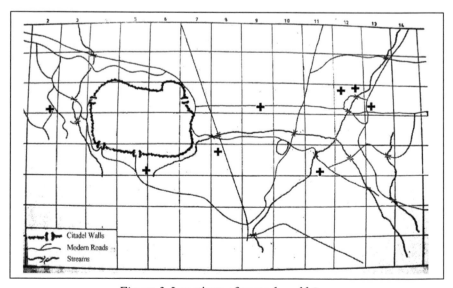

Figure 3. Locations of some *bozakhānes*

Kocanaib: column 2; Pınarbaşı: col. 5; Tahtakale: col. 8; Gallebazarı col. 9; Sedbaşı: col. 11; Kanberler: col. 12; Atbazarı: col. 12; Tatarlar: col. 13[12]

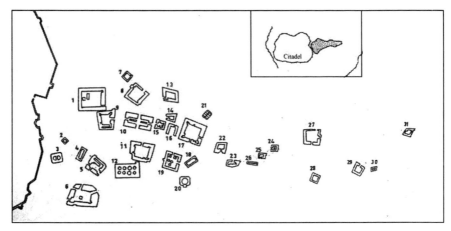

Figure 4. Locations of commercial centers and public buildings

1. Pirinç Hanı, 2. Balı Bey Hanı, 3. Çakır Ağa Hamamı, 4. Doğan Gözü Hanı, 5. Kapan Hanı, 6. Bayezid Paşa Hanı, 7. Kuşbazlar Hanı, 8. Karacabey Hanı, 9. Harir Hanı, 10. Bedestan, 11. Emir Hanı, 12. Ulucami, 13. Eski Yeni Hanı, 14. Sandıkçılar Hanı, 15. Gevye Hanı, 16. Yeni Harir Hanı, 17. Mahmud Paşa Hanı, 18. Han Remnants, 19. Koza Hanı, 20. Orhan Camii, 21. Yolgeçen Odaları, 22. Bezir Hanı, 23. Tuz Hanı, 24. Hacı Osman Hanı, 25. Kütahya Hanı, 26. Han Remnants, 27. Yeni Tahıl Hanı, 28. Han Remnants, 29. Han Remnants, 30. Han Remnants, 31. Kanberler Hanı.[13]

The old Gallebazarı (also known as Tahılbazarı, the cereal market) and its *han* (commercial inn) were near the Tuzhanı (wholesale salt market) built in the fifteenth century. Until the reign of Süleyman the Magnificent (r. 1520–66), this district was among the most active commercial centers of the town. The Gallebazarı *bozakhāne* must have been located in this commercial district during the late fifteenth century.[14]

During the late fifteenth century, the area comprising the *leblebiciler çarşısı* (the market of the sellers of roasted chick peas), and Tahtakale known as Eski Çarşı located near the cereal market, were at the heart of commercial life. Streets full of workshops and retail stores of craftsmen, such as *haffāf*s (shoemakers) and the Han of Bayezid Paşa, as well as a *bozakhāne* existed in Tahtakale.[15] With the later shift of the commercial district towards the east, during Süleyman's reign, this part of town acquired the name *eski* (old).

Atbazarı (the horse market), where the Atbazarı *bozakhāne* was established, was near the so-called Tatarlar neighborhood, although there is no clear evidence that the inhabitants of this district were actually Tatars.[16] Kanberler *bozakhāne* was in the Kanberler neighborhood (to the west of the Tatarlar Bridge), which developed around the mosque built by Sitti Hatun in 1456.[17] This district is known to have turned into a wealthy area only in the late sixteenth century; therefore a century earlier compared to the area around Uzunçarşı (the central long market) it was among the less commercial parts of the town.[18] The Pınarbaşı neighborhood and *bozakhāne* were in the southwestern edge of the citadel, near the neighborhood of Alaca Hırka. One of the water sources of the city originated there and reached the tannery and Tahtakale, which made Pınarbaşı a crucial center for its immediate surrounding area.[19]

Having looked at the locations of the *bozakhāne*s of Bursa, one wonders what kind of economic value each *bozakhāne* carried in its heyday. A systematic analysis of two collections (*defter*s) of Bursa court records (*sicil*s) informs us about the *boza* business in Bursa. *Defter* A-4 (1484) comprises a total of 6,914 documents, fifty of which concern *bozakhāne*s; whereas *defter* A-8 (1490–91) comprises a total of 6,849 court cases, ninety-three of which involve *bozakhāne*s. These may seem to be small numbers in relation to the total of the seven hundred and thirty-four documents that relate to artisans and state intervention in economic affairs found in just one *defter* (A-8), yet the *bozakhāne* trade is the most frequently mentioned in *defter* A8; the next most frequently mentioned are the dyers (*sabbāğ*) of silk textiles, appearing in seventy-two records.

*Defter*s A-4 and A-8 reveal that as of 1484 all *bozakhāne*s of Bursa remained active, with the addition of seven new ones by 1491.[20] Relevant information that can be found in these records includes the name of the *bozakhāne*, the name of the tenant (*müste'cir*) to whom the *bozakhāne* was rented (*bozakhāne dutan*), the months and dates or the duration of the rental period, the amount paid, the names of the official supervisors with financial and administrative responsibilities (*emīn, āmil, kātib,* or *cābī*), the names of the agents, representatives, witnesses, and the deputy of the *qadi* (*kefīl, vekīl, şāhid,* or *nāib*) as well as, in some cases, specific details concerning legal transactions. In sum, court cases mostly reflect fiscal operations involving the rents and taxes extracted from *bozakhāne*s. While they provide limited information on the social interactions that took place in these establishments, they shed light on the question of how individual *bozakhāne*s compare to each other.

In this framework, I observe that the *bozakhāne* of the Balıkbazarı neighborhood, which was mostly inhabited by Greeks after the Ottoman conquest, is the one appearing most frequently in *defter*s A-4 and A-8 in a total of twenty-four cases. This *bozakhāne* had the highest rent, towering at one hundred *akçe*s per day. The other *bozakhāne*s appear between one and thirteen times each, with an average of ten cases.[21] Two *bozakhāne*s that appear thirteen times each are those in Gallebazarı and Odalar, which are both commercial neighborhoods.[22] Gallebazarı is also among the *bozakhāne*s with the highest rent. This situation may lead to the assumption that the popularity of a *bozakhāne* and the rent it paid were correlated to its proximity to commercial districts.

*Bozakhāne*s functioned on state-owned (*mīrī*) property. Therefore a fee (*resm*) was extracted from each one. Tax officials (*āmil, emīn,* or *mültezim*) were in charge of collecting the fee and sending it to the treasury, or in the case of Bursa, to the imperial agent for palace purchases (*khassa kharc emīni*).[23] A closer examination of the identity, authority, terms of engagement, and various functions of the tax officials illustrates the relationship between the fiscal and administrative aspects of state involvement in the *boza* business.

What do court records tell us about the people involved in the *boza* business? As far as state officials are concerned, court cases reveal that the *emīn* was the person who managed a specific source of tax revenue.[24] He collected the *bozakhāne* payments (*rüsūm*), which consisted of two parts, one being the down payment (*yevm'ül-kıst*) taken in advance by the *emīn* toward the agreed upon maximum annual rent of the *bozakhāne*. For instance the *yevm'ül-kıst* of a *bozakhāne* could be 90 *akçe*s for a month and a half, which meant that the annual rent was 60 times 12, or 720 *akçe*s. The amount of the *yevm'ül-kıst* was always specified and allows us to calculate the annual rent of *bozakhāne*s whenever this information is available. The second part of the payment was called *resm-i kitābet* and was collected at the time of signing the contract, as a registration fee.

The contract was signed between the tax official (*emīn*) and the tenant (*müste'cīr*). In a court case that illustrates payments collected from *boza-*

khānes, it is related that Seydi Ahmed b. Resul, who was the *emīn* of Bursa *bozkhānes*, came to the *qadi* court saying that he received exactly 20,645 *akças* as *bozakhāne* payments from the tenant of the Balıkbazarı *bozakhāne*, Ali b. Abdullah. The same record also specifies that the previous *emīn* of *bozkhānes*, who was appointed by the *qadi,* said that he had formerly taken a month and a half's worth of the rent from the same tenant.[25] No complaint or conflict exists in this case; rather, it is a record kept for notarial purposes.

A case from *defter* A-8 reads as follows:

> Mustafa Çelebi son of Mehmed, who had been appointed *emīn* to the *bozakhānes* of Bursa by the *qadi,* said the following at the *qadi* court: 'When I was appointed as *emīn*, the tenant Hacı Ali delivered to me the *bozakhāne* payments of the Tahıl Bazarı (Galle Bazarı) *bozakhāne* for a month and a half, from the fifteenth of Receb till the last day of Şā'ban in the year 895 (May 30–July 19, 1490). Witnesses: Mevlānā Eyüb, Mevlana Sinan el-Katib, Yahya b. Mehmed, and Hızır b. Abdullah.[26]

In another case from the same *defter,* it is related that the tax official of Bursa *bozakhānes*, Mehmed b. Seydī Ya'kūb, sold the estate of a *boza* maker who had disappeared without paying his rent: "*Boza* maker Hacı Ali son of Yaya (Baba?) Ali, who was renting [a *bozakhāne*] under my supervision had the remainder of the *bozakhāne* rent on him when he disappeared without paying it. Mevlānā Kestellü [the *qadi*] ordered his estate to be sold. I sold the estate of the aforementioned with the help of Mustafa Çelebi, who was sent by the *qadi* to summon Hacı Ali. I took the full payment received for the estate (1,010 *akçes*) from the wife of the *boza* maker, Ayşe bint-i Ramazan. Witnesses: Mevlānā Mehmed b. 'Ali el-..., Mevlānā Muslihiddīn b. Hasan, Mevlānā Seydī el-Hatīb, and the scribe of the written words."[27]

The *muqātā'a* system of taxation, records of which we have seen above, was not only a fiscal practice, but also, and perhaps more significantly, an administrative one. We learn from sultanic law codes (*qanunnāmes*) that the centrally issued diplomas (*berāts*) of *emīns* (or *mültezims*) equipped them with the right and responsibility not only of tax collection, but also the supervision of the relationships among the people involved in the revenue-generating activity (such as weighing silk textiles in the case of the silk industry). [28] The tax collector was therefore both a member of the administrative (*'örf/'urf*) sphere and an economic agent. [29] Diplomas determined the terms of tax collection and gave directions on how to administer the activities of Ottoman subjects (*re'āyā*) in a particular sphere of activity. *Emīn*s (or *mültezim*s) were often appointed based on the testimony of guarantors who appeared in the *qadi* court. This testimony attested both the property and the integrity (*kefīl-i bi'l-māl ve kefīl-i bi'n-nefs*) of the candidate for the office. The testimony regarding the character/personality of the tax official included evidence of his moral strength, piety, and honesty. In turn, he was given the right to expect the same level of integrity and honesty from those who worked for him.

From the government's point of view, the administrative functions of the *emīn* included the choice of the physical place where a *bozakhāne* was to be established. The majority of *bozakhāne* buildings of fifteenth-century Bursa were owned by the state, and supervised by an *emīn*. In addition to renting the physical space, one of the duties of the *emīn* was to choose the tenant-managers of the *bozakhāne*s from among a pool of applicants. The *emīn* preferred higher-paying tenants, but the ideal moral character required of the *emīn* by the state must also have applied to his choice of the tenants.

The clerk (*bozakhāne kātibi*) was the person who kept the records related to the *bozakhāne*s. The following court case relates that Mustafa b. Mehmed, who was appointed *bozakhāne* scribe by the principal tax official (*āmil*), was paid 388 *akçe*s in return for his services for a duration of three and a half months in 1496. The amount of 388 for three and a half months means he had a daily wage of four *akçe*s. [30] He received this amount from the tax farmer, with the permission of the principal tax farmer. Clearly, the hiring and salary of the clerk were approved by the highest authority in the particular sphere of activity related to that tax source. The aforementioned case suggests that the government contracted the running of *boza muqāta'a* to a principal tax farmer (*'āmil*) who subcontracted part of it to another contractor (*emīn*). In this respect, this practice cannot be interpreted merely as a reflection of increased state control, but rather as a more complex structure of delegation of powers by contractors and subcontractors. The existence of tax farmers as well as a principal tax farmer implies a hierarchy among them, thus indicating increased bureaucratization and central control over tax collection in the period in question.

The names of the *bozakhāne* managers (or tenants) show that they hailed from various backgrounds and denominations. A number of them were probably former slaves or converts as can be understood from the patronymic, "son of Abdullah" (ibn Abdullah) attached to their names, for example Ali b. Abdullah, Karagöz b. Abdullah, İlyas b. Abdullah, and Yusuf b. Abdullah—a feature that is fairly common in fifteenth-century Bursa records due to a lively slave market, extensive local use of slave labor, and the subsequent conversion of these individuals to Islam.[31] Furthermore, some tenants' names are among those customarily given to converts, such as Karagöz, Elvan, and Babam geldi/güldi. One of them is registered as "Arab Oğlu Azadlusı Karagöz b. Abdullah" (Karagöz, the former slave of the Son of Arab).[32] There are two tenants whose names are Emek and Guri, indicating they might be non-Muslims. Another one is "Tatar Süleyman b. Ali." Many, however, appear to be Muslim born.

A minority of the *bozakhāne* tenants' names (twenty-eight out of one hundred and forty-three cases on *bozakhāne*s) include epithets or nicknames suggesting an association with a trade or ethnic group. *Bozā ʾī* (*boza* maker in Arabic, which is the language used in the majority of the fifteenth-century court records) appears in nine cases. Seven are marked as freed slaves, one as a slave, five as *hacı* (A. *alhāj* / O. *elhāc*: in this context: merchant and not pilgrim), and three as both *bozacı* (*boza* maker in Turkish) and *hacı*. Both court records and other sources refer to Tatars and Albanians as ethnic groups who were especially involved in the *boza* business. As a matter of fact, Tatar *bozası* was banned in Bursa at different periods due to its excessive alcohol content. More will be said below about the moral concerns of the Ottoman government regarding the *boza* business.

From the fiscal and administrative points of view, the main concern of the legal court was to establish and register the duration of the rental contract (which varied between one and twelve months) and the amount of the agreed upon rent. As previously mentioned, the rents paid for the Balıkbazarı, Gallebazarı, Atbazarı, Kanber, Tahtakale, and Yeni (also located in Tahtakale) *bozakhāne*s, which were mostly located in highly commercial districts, were the highest. While the rent of each *bozakhāne* varied over time, the rental values of *bozakhāne*s relative to each other seem to have remained constant. The records point to a downward trend in the *bozakhāne* rents between 1484 and 1491. The daily rent of the Balıkbazarı *bozakhāne* appears to have declined from one hundred to seventy *akçe*s between 1484 and 1491; that of the Gallebazarı *bozakhāne* from ninety to forty *akçe*s within the same period; that of the Kanber *bozakhāne* from eighty to thirty-one; and that of the Tahtakale *bozakhāne* from sixty-five to eighteen.[33]

Apart from daily rents, some lump-sum figures are also recorded with vague descriptions such as *"Brusa'daki bozakhānelerden"* (collected from the *bozakhāne*s in Bursa). These sums, approximately ranging from twenty thousand to forty thousand *akçe*s, were usually collected from various *bozakhāne*s for the expenditures of the imperial agent for palace purchases *(khassa kharc emīni)*. For example, in a document dated May 9, 1491, it is recorded that "Sadreddin b. Hüdadad, the imperial agent for palace purchases in Bursa, came to the *qadi* court and said that he took 22,600 *akçe*s from the *bozakhāne* income by the order of the principal tax farmer Salih b. Yusuf, from the hands of the tax farmer Seydi Ahmed b. Resul, in order to pay for *khassa kharcı* expenses."[34]

Court cases mentioning lump-sum figures give no detail on the duration of the rental period. Nevertheless they raise the question of how *bozakhāne* rents were actually changed. In 1492, *boza*-makers came to the court demanding a decrease in their *bozakhāne* rents due to an epidemic that emerged in Bursa. Their request was granted to bring about the following reduction in rents:[35]

TABLE 2

Varying Bozakhāne Rents (1492)

Bozakhāne	Old Rent (in *akçe*)	New Rent (in *akçe*)
Balıkbazarı	80	65
Gallebazarı	50	40
Odalar	31	25
Sedbaşı	50	30
Pınarbaşı	25	16
Yeni	40	30
Tahtakale	42	25
Tatarlar	Unchanged (*asıl üzre*)	

We find a bit more detail in a parallel case from the previous year. The case relates that Hacı Mehmed b. Abdullah, who held the Kabluca *bozakhāne* for ten *akçe*s a day with his partner, quit the operation, claiming that business was slow ("*çok iş itmezüz deyū bıraġub vaz gelmiş idi*"). After the *bozakhāne* remained vacant for a few days, Hacı Mehmed re-rented it for five *akçe*s a day.[36] Another document indicates that in the following days the rents of several *bozakhāne*s were lowered due to slow business: the Balıkbazarı *bozakhāne* in the hands of Ali (from eighty to seventy *akçe*s a day) and the Çakıllu *bozakhāne* run by Hüseyin (from twelve to seven *akçe*s a day).[37]

Hasan Basri Öcalan has documented a comparable situation in 1515, when some *bozakhāne* holders applied for a reduction of their rents due to slow business. The court approved this request, and the rents of Gallebazarı, Tatarlar, Yeni, Kanberler, Kayabaşı, Kocanaib, and Tahtakale *bozakhāne*s, were reduced.[38] Öcalan's research also shows that a similar reduction took place in 1518, as indicated in the following chart:[39]

TABLE 3

Reduction in Bozakhāne Rents (1518)

Bozakhāne	Old Rent (in *akçe*)	New rent (in *akçe*)
Balıkbazarı	55	42
Gallebazarı	45	35
Sedbaşı	25	8
Tahtakale	30	20
Yeni	58	43
Kayabaşı	30	20
Tatarlar	50	40

Rent reductions were by no means the only change that took place. Rents sometimes increased through competition. For example in 1492, one Hacı Mustafa b. Mehmed managed to take the Kabluca *bozakhāne* away from Salih b. Yusuf, who was paying four *akçe*s a day, by offering to pay a daily rent of sixteen *akçe*s.[40] But soon after, Salih offered eight more *akçe*s and took back his *bozakhāne*. In this competition, Salih went from paying a daily rent that was four *akçe*s up to a rent of twenty-four *akçe*s within a few days.[41] These cases confirm that the state's agents (*emīn/mültezim*) preferred tenants who were able to offer higher rents, which also explains how *bozakhāne*s changed hands. However, the fiscal matters were not the only aspect of the *boza* business that concerned the Ottoman government.

Outside the Fiscal Sphere:
Bozakhāne as a Point of Public Interaction,
Entertainment and Crime

Some other characteristics of *boza* and its consumption that attracted the attention of the government included the alcohol content of the fermented drink, the public character of *bozakhāne*s, and the heterogeneity of their clientele. The government perceived Ottoman society as divided into easily recognizable units called *tā'ife* (A. class, sect, body of people, denomination) or *cemā'at* (A. band, community, assembly, congregation). Whether the term referred to religious, occupational, or ethnic groups, *tā'ife*s possessed a certain degree of autonomy under the leadership and supervision of a steward (*ketkhüdā*). This autonomy ideally meant that the members' collective will prevailed within each group. The government perceived the *ketkhüdā* both as the representative of the *tā'ife* and as an extension of the central authority. While one cannot assume that both functions were of equal significance for the holder of the position, circumstances dictated which one of these two functions held the greatest importance at any given moment. *Tā'ife*s, which were religiously, ethnically, or professionally homogenous groups, might have exercised greater autonomy in the formative period of the Ottoman power. With centralization well on its way by the mid-fifteenth century, the same groups are likely to have felt the increasing presence of the state. Yet even at the height of centralization and imperial power, these local associations of people remained at least partially autonomous, and the relationship they enjoyed with government authorities deserves a closer look.

In an urban setting, public places such as bathhouses, winehouses, and *boza* houses are known to have brought together individuals from various backgrounds, therefore creating heterogeneous groups of patrons. People of different occupations, diverse religions and ethnicities, and various neighborhoods, whether from the rural hinterland, another town, or a distant foreign land, could gather in a *bozakhāne*. While rules that set behavioral possibilities or limits for individuals within homogeneous groups were overseen by their respective stewards, a higher legal and political authority seems to have organized the rules of the "intermediary sphere" where people of heterogeneous identities came together.

Court cases show that the consumption of sour, highly fermented, and thus alcoholic *ekşi boza* created tensions that became a serious source of concern for government authorities. In this respect, the government sought the best possible tax farmer to pick the best possible tenant, who would prevent the sale of alcoholic *boza*. With moral integrity and honesty being among the tax official's concerns, it was not uncommon for him to request guarantors who would testify not only to the financial solvency (*kefīl-i bi'l-māl*) but also the good character of the tenant (*kefīl-i bi'n-nefs*). Since the *bozakhāne* tax was one of the most lucrative enterprises for the government, the tenant had to be able to make regular payments, hence the requirement of guarantors of his financial status (*kefīl-i bi'l-māl*). Yet the intention to secure a tenant who was both financially and morally sound, may have been rarely, if ever, fulfilled in reality.

Another dimension of the government's interest in public places such as *bozakhāne*s was the diversity of the backgrounds of their patrons. Merchants, wandering dervishes, folk poets, story-tellers (*meddāh*), and foreign travelers could socialize in the same *bozakhāne*. Considering the technological limitations of the time, these individuals were significant agents of communication. They not only exchanged news and passed on information, but also added their own perspectives, comments, and spin to the stories they related. Merchants engaged in long-distance trade were significant actors in this respect, thus the Ottoman government took the possibility of political and social criticism occurring in *bozakhane*s seriously—keeping the ownership of the facilities, and keeping detailed records of their administration through state-appointed agents.[42]

There was always the possibility that spontaneous debates or disputes in public places would take on a political character and spread throughout the town. Such political debates generally came in some religious guise, and therefore only this religious aspect might be readily recognizable. Still, the government had considerable interest in keeping such public places under some, but by no means absolute, control for the sake of political stability. One might, for example, overhear the expression of a nascent opposition movement in a *bozakhāne*, although praise for the state could have also been heard. A few people could be engaged in a casual friendly conversation (*sohbet*), while a larger group listened to the songs and poems of a folk poet (*āşık*) or popular chants about various Ottoman cities. These performances did not only entertain but might contain satirical, even critical commentaries and therefore rendered the *bozakhāne*s worthy of the government's attention.

This potential of the *boza* houses as places that would facilitate political opposition and social criticism was not the only feature that attracted the government's attention. They were also places where entertainment could breach morally tolerable limits, which the government felt obliged to observe to maintain its image of legitimacy.

Scholarly literature on leisure activities during the classical Ottoman period mostly focuses on the well-documented festivities organized by the royal family, for occasions such as imperial weddings, births and circumcisions of princes, and grand banquets. This literature falls short of informing us about the leisure activities of ordinary people.[43] A notable exception in this respect is the work of Fikret Yılmaz. He relies on sixteenth-century court records to develop a useful approach to understand entertainment patterns of ordinary people in Ottoman times.[44] According to Yılmaz's findings the leisure activities of ordinary people ranged from Ramazan and religious holiday celebrations, to javelin games, to the promotion ceremonies of artisans, to weddings, and to festivals that took place at picnic grounds.

Yılmaz makes a conceptual distinction between leisure activities that served a larger purpose of a public nature for their organizers and leisure activities that were relatively private affairs. Thus, imperial celebrations helped legitimize the dynasty and political authority. Meetings organized by artisans and Sufi orders helped reinforce the internal solidarity and hierarchy of the respective groups. Marriage festivals sanctioned the union of the newlyweds while also reflecting the place of their families in the society. Religious festivities reinforced beliefs and community spirit. Harvest

festivals generated local and often inter-religious connections while celebrating the bounties of nature. More private activities, on the other hand,
were born out of the personal preferences and the will of small groups and
did not involve the initiative of a higher authority or elders.[45]

These two types of leisure activities are documented through two different sets of sources. Public activities included poetic texts describing imperial weddings, banquets or circumcision festivals (*sürnāme*s), miniatures,
courtly *dīvān* poetry, travel accounts, and the records of palace expenditures. A different and less systematic set of sources offers information on
private activities, especially with respect to leisure activity that took place
on the outskirts of Istanbul and other towns. These latter sources include
court registers, popular literature including poems written about towns, and
travel accounts. Fifteenth-century Bursa court records provide significant
information on the fiscal and economic aspects of *bozakhāne*s, but shed
rather indirect and limited light on the entertainment of their patrons. We
can, however, benefit from research on other towns or on Bursa from later
periods to imagine these activities and hope to refine our understanding of
the aspects of *bozakhāne*s outside of their fiscal and economic sides, if and
when richer information becomes available to us eventually.

We know from Yılmaz's work on nearby Edremit that eating and drinking (*yiyip içme*) went hand in hand with friendly conversation (a crucial
component of leisure and entertainment) and might edge into a realm that
would be considered "criminal" by legal norms of the period.[46] The drink
in question in these situations was mostly wine (but occasionally *rakı*) in
the sixteenth century.[47] Where would the activities of the *bozakhāne* stand
in this continuum where entertainment verged on crime? The answer re-
volves around the legal statues of *boza* as a beverage. Some legal scholars
considered it intoxicating and therefore forbidden while others claimed it
was permissible. Berthold Laufer suggests a connection between *boza* and
the English word *booze*, although he cautions the reader to distinguish between the noun *booze* and the verb *to booze*, which has a Germanic origin.[48]
Quite a few travelogues from different periods include references to the intoxicating nature of *boza*, and it appears that the word sometimes had the
meaning of a "drinking-bout." One such account appears in the nineteenth-
century Swiss traveler and Orientalist J. L. Burckhardt's *Travels in Nubia*:

Few traders pass through Berber without taking a mistress, if it be only for a fortnight. Drunkenness is the constant companion of this debauchery, and it would seem as if the men in these countries had no other objects in life. The intoxicating liquor, which they drink is called *buza*. Strongly leavened bread made from dhurra [sorghum] is broken into crumbs, and mixed with water, and the mixture is kept for several hours over a slow fire. Being then removed, water is poured over it, and it is left for two nights to ferment. This liquor, according to its greater or smaller degree of fermentation, takes the names of *merin*, or *buza*, or *om belbel*, the mother of nightingales, so called because it makes the drunkard sing.[49]

The Islamic ban on alcohol finds its roots in the Qur'ān, where the first reference appears in Sūra II, 219: "They will ask thee about intoxicants and games of chance. Say: 'In both there is great evil as well as some benefit for man; but the evil which they cause is greater than the benefit which they bring.'"[50] Sūra IV, 43, which was revealed at a later date, suggested that drinking may be enervating to the point of losing consciousness: "O you who have attained to faith! Do not attempt to pray while you are in a state of drunkenness, [but wait] until you know what you are saying."[51] Another revelation (Sūra V, 90–91) established the definitive prohibition: "O you who have attained to faith! Intoxicants, and games of chance, and idolatrous practices, and the divining of the future are but a loathsome evil of Satan's doing: shun it, then, so that you might attain a happy state! By means of intoxicants and games of chance Satan seeks only to sow enmity and hatred among you, and to turn you away from the rememberance of God and from prayer. Will you not, then, resist?"[52]

Islamic law prohibits not only the consumption, but also the public display of wine consumption both for Muslims and non-Muslims. This was deemed a crime committed against God and therefore was subject to the *khadd* punishment. The market inspector (*muhtasib*) or other designated officials punished the flagrant offenders. In fact, rather than the actual act of drinking wine, what really concerned the *muhtasib* was the display of this act in public places (*idh'hār*).[53] As much as the prohibition of wine was clear in the Qur'ānic verses, the extension of this principle to other alcoholic drinks needed further legal elaboration. As a fermented drink, *boza* was thus liable to be prohibited, especially when it was sold and consumed publicly.

Another significant characteristic of *bozakhāne*s was the possibility that they could serve wine upon request, giving authorities an additional reason for placing them under surveillance. Depending on the duration of fermentation, the alcohol content in *boza* could reach levels sufficiently high enough to intoxicate an adult. Ottoman authorities thus distinguished between *tatlı* (sweet and permissible) and *ekşi boza* (sour, alcoholic, and forbidden).[54] A Bursa court case from 1583 describes a woman who came to the court claiming that her husband had sworn an oath not to drink wine or sour *boza* (*ekşi boza*), or else he would divorce her.[55] The consumption of alcoholic *boza* was not permissible for the Muslim population, especially in public places like the *bozakhāne*s. It was also banned for non-Muslims, however, probably because of the difficulty in distinguishing between Muslim and non-Muslim patrons.

Seventeenth-century Bursa court records cited by Hasan Basri Öcalan also highlight the association of drinking, especially *boza* consumption, with crime, confirming the evidence put forward by Fikret Yılmaz based on the *sicil*s of Edremit. In 1614, a group of Muslims were discovered with a pitcher of sour *boza* in the Hamzabey quarter, having fun in the company of two women named Rāziye and Sāliha.[56] In 1630, when the sharp rise in popularity of the coffeehouses was well under way, Bursa wine-houses and *bozakhāne*s were banned from selling wine and *boza* and were temporarily closed down before the Ramadan celebrations. On the second day of the religious holiday, however, a group of ruffians broke the locks on the doors of one of the closed establishments, opened the wine casks, and started partying with the women they brought along with them disguised in men's clothes. They then wounded a soldier and fled. Subsequently the court sent armed officers after them. The next day they were brought to the court but then ran away with one of the female detainees.[57] Bursa *bozakhāne*s were occasionally closed as a result of complaints specifically about alcohol consumption in them. In such a case from 1671, the plaintiff said: "We are unable to go out (of our houses) because of the *boza* drunks. Mischief-makers filled up our town."[58]

The seventeenth-century Ottoman traveler Evliya Çelebi, who visited Bursa in 1640, offers the following account of Bursa's *bozakhāne*s:

There are also no less than ninety-seven *bozakhāne*s, which are not to be equaled in the world; they are wainscoted with faience, painted, each capable of accommodating one thousand men. In summer *boza* is cooled in ice, like sherbet; the principal men of the town are not ashamed to enter these *bozakhāne*s, although an abundance of youths, dancers and singers, wrapped in Bursa girdles here entice their lovers to ruin.[59]

Upon entering a *bozakhāne* in Ankara, Evliya Çelebi claims to have been bothered by what he perceived as an environment of moral laxity and casual entertainment, and soon he decided to leave.[60] Leaving aside Evliya Çelebi's habit of inflating the numbers, his characterization of the *bozakhāne*s as public places seems quite plausible.

An example of the connection between eating and intoxicating drinks appears in a court case from seventeenth-century Istanbul, which reveals an interesting claim put forward by *boza* makers (*bozacı*): The *bozacı*s claimed that sautéed liver (*ciğer kebabı*) was their exclusive specialty by long established custom. Therefore, no one else could sell it, unlike meatballs (*köfte*) and other similar dishes, which could be made and sold by other tradesmen such as cooks and kebab makers.[61] If the liver kebab was as popular an accompaniment of alcoholic drinks in the seventeenth century as it is today, the *bozacı*s' exclusive claim to the right of serving it could imply that *bozakhāne*s were public places where people went "to eat and drink" and get drunk in the seventeenth century Istanbul.[62]

Conclusion

In this paper I outlined certain aspects of the *bozakhāne*s of late fifteenth-century Bursa, where the popular fermented *boza* drink was made and sold. The figures on *bozakhāne* rents back in late fifteenth-century Bursa examined above indicate that the Bursa *bozakhāne*s were significant sources of revenue for the government. The magnitude of these figures suggests that *bozakhāne*s engaged not merely in the production and house-to-house distribution of the drink, but also in its retail sale. Moreover, since *boza* was a drink that had to be served fresh, it could not be kept for long periods in storage places in containers like wine casks. This peculiarity of *boza* strengthens the possibility that not only the *bozakhāne*s mentioned by Evliyā Çelebi, but also the earlier ones resembled taverns open to the public. *Bozakhāne* locations suggested a relationship between their rents and their proximity to commercial districts. A comparison of Bursa court records of later periods and those from some other Ottoman towns by Hasan Basri Öcalan and Fikret Yılmaz indicate a strong association between eating, drinking, and alcoholic *boza* consumption, which was yet another factor that placed *boza* affairs under the special scrutiny of the government.

*Bozakhāne*s, where immoral and criminal activities have been recorded by the court registers, seem to have retained their popularity until the rise of the coffeehouses in Ottoman towns in the seventeenth century. The seventeenth-century triumph of the coffeehouse over other public places such as *bozakhāne*s suggests the popularity of caffeine over other mood-changing/altering substances.

Notes

1. Bursa Court Records (BCR) A-8 670: 9 Cumāde'l-evvel, 896. March 20, 1491: *Brūsa bozakhānelerinde emīn olan Seydi Ahmed b. Resul şer'iyyat mahfelinde iqrār idüb eyitdi ki Kanber bozakhānesin dutan İlyas b. Abdullah elinden zikr olan bozakhānenin yevm'ül-qıstı ve resm-i kitābeti bī küsūr sene sitte ve tıs'īn ve semānemi'e rebiyülevvel ġurresinden sene-yi mezkūre rebiyy'ül-ākhiri ġāyetine varınca baña vāsıl oldı didi ol dakhī tasdīk itdi. ŞH: Mustafa b. Mehmed; Mevlana Eyüb; ve kātib'ül-khurūf; ve Mevlana Sinan el-Din.*

2. The *boza* drink is known to have been consumed and enjoyed in the Crimea, the Balkans, the Middle East, and North Africa. Various hypotheses have been put forward about the origins of the word *boza*, possibly of ancient Turkish origin, which seems to have passed onto Slavic and Western languages. While Steingass records this word as Persian, in Vambery it is listed as an ancient Turkish word, which is also found in *Kutadgu Bilig*. The word was adopted in the form of *bodzo* by the Mongols. The Ottoman version is recorded by Th. Smith of Oxford in 1674 in the *Epistola de moribus ac insitutis Turcarum* as "They also have other liquors rather peculiar to them of which I shall only mention *Bozza* made from millet." Lane mentions *boozeh* or *boozah* as a drink that was popular among the boatmen of the Nile and other people of the lower

ranks of society. From Ottoman, the word has passed on to Slavic and Balkan languages, French, Spanish, Portugese, etc. See Berthold Laufer, "On the Possible Oriental Origin of Our Word Booze," *Journal of the American Oriental Society* 49 (1929): p. 58.

3. Balıkbazarı, Sedbaşı, Gallebazarı, Tahtakale, Atbazarı, and Odalar.

4. Kanberler and Çakıllı *bozakhāne*s. See Hasan Basri Öcalan, "Bursa'da Boza ve Tarihi Bozahaneler," in *I. Bursa Halk Kültürü Sempozyumu Bildiri Kitabı*, ed. Y. Oğuzoğlu and K. Üstünova (Bursa: Bursa University Press, 2002), vol. 1, p. 117.

5. Kapluca, Yeni Bozakhāne, Pınarbaşı, Tatarlar, Kocanaib, Yenikapı, and Sultan Hatun Odaları.

6. Özer Ergenç, *XVI. Yüzyılın Sonlarında Bursa: Yerleşimi, Yönetimi, Ekonomik ve Sosyal Durumu Üzerine bir Araştırma* (Ankara: Türk Tarih Kurumu, 2006), p. 120.

7. To the districts of Kayabaşı, Demirkapı, Balıkbazarı, Kuruçeşme, Sedbaşı, and Karaağaç (near Kayabaşı). Bursa court records show that among the non-Muslims, Armenians were settled in Sedbaşı; Greeks in Balıkbazarı, Kayabaşı and Demirkapı; and Jews in Kuruçeşme.

8. Maps and illustrations were prepared by Özer Ergenç and are here reprinted with the permission of the author. I am greatly indebted to him for providing me with copies of these illustrations and the corresponding lists of neighborhoods prior to their publication in his book on sixteenth-century Bursa: Özer Ergenç, *XVI. Yüzyılın Sonlarında Bursa* (Ankara: Turk Tarih Kurumu, 2006). I located and marked some of the districts with *bozakhāne*s on these illustrations, insofar as it is possible to determine the locations of the *bozakhāne*s based on the limited information we have at this point.

9. Ergenç, *Bursa*, pp. 325–28.

10. Ergenç. *Bursa*, pp. 325–28.

11. Ergenç, *Bursa*, pp. 325–28.

12. Based on the map of Bursa in Ergenç, *Bursa*, Appendix, pp. 325–28.

13. Ergenç, *Bursa*, pp. 325–28.

14. Ergenç, *Bursa*, p. 29.

15. Ergenç, *Bursa*, p. 30.

16. This neighborhood, also called the Tatar Hace district roughly corresponds to the Kurtuluş Mahallesi in modern day Bursa. Ergenç, *Bursa*, p. 61.

17. Kazım Baykal, *Bursa ve Anıtları* (Bursa: Eski Eserleri Sevenler Kurumu, 1950), p. 129.

18. Ergenç, *Bursa, pp.* 27–28.

19. Ergenç, *Bursa*, p. 47.

20. Located in (and in most cases named after) the neighborhoods of Pınarbaşı, Kapluca, Yeni Bozakhāne (also located in Tahtakale) Sultan Hatun Odaları, Yenikapı, Tatarlar and Kocanaib.

21. Odalar and Gallebazarı (thirteen times each), Tahtakale and Kapluca (twelve times each), Yeni Bozakhāne and Kanber ([Kanberler]-eleven times each), Çakıllı (nine times), Pınarbaşı (eight times), Tatarlar (seven times), Atbazarı (six times), Kocanaib (two times) and Sultan Hatun Odaları (once).

22. One can suppose that Odalar (lit. the "rooms") refer to bachelors' residences that commonly hosted craftsmen working in this commercial district.

23. On this official, see: Halil Inalcık, "Bursa XV. Asır Sanayi ve Ticaret Tarihine Dair Vesikalar," *Belleten* 24 (1960): pp. 45–102; Özer Ergenç, "Osmanlı Klasik Döneminde İstanbul'un Statüsü ve Yönetimi" (Paper delivered at the İstanbul'un Fethi ve Fatih Sempozyumu, İstanbul 14–15 Haziran 2003). See also Ergenç, *Bursa*; and Arif Bilgin, *Osmanlı Taşrasında bir Maliye Kurumu: Bursa Hassa Harç Eminliği* (Istanbul: Kitabevi, 2006).

24. *Muqāt'ayı der-uhde iden*: *muqātā'a* was the right to collect the taxes and fees from a specified source of revenue.

25. BCR A-8/1287: 28 Cumāde'l-ākhire 896. May 8, 1491. "Brūsa boza-hānelerinde emīn olan Seydi Ahmed b. Resul şer'iyat mahfelinde ikrār idüb eyitdi ki: Balık bazarı bozakhānesin dutan Ali b. Abdullah elinden zikr olan bozahāneniñ yevmü'l-kıstı ve resm-i kitābetin sene hamse ne tis'īn semānemi'e Şevvāl ġurresinden sene sitte ve tis'īn semānemi'e Cumāde'l-evveli ākherine varınca yiğrmi biñ altıyüz kırkbeş akça bī kusūr alub kabz eyledim didi oldakhī tasdīk ve sābıkan qadi tarafından emīn olan Tuli Çelebi dakhī ikrār idüb eyitdi ki: zikr olan bozahāneniñ yevmü'l-kıst ve resm-i kitābet sene hamse ve tis'a ve semānemi'e Recebinin nısfından Şa'bān ākherine varınca ki bir buçuk aylıkdır bī kusūr mezkūr Ali elinden alub kabz eledüm didi. ŞH: Mevlana Bali b. Ivaz; ve Musa b. Hasan; ve Mevlana Eyüb; ve Ahmed b. Abdullah."

26. BCR A-8/682.

27. BCR A-8/665.

28. Nicoară Beldiceanu, *Recherche sur la Ville Ottomane au xve Siecle: Etude et Actes* (Paris: Librairie d'amérique et d'orient Adrien Maisonneuve, 1953), pp. 68–71. Please note that in the late fifteenth century *emīn*s and *mültezim*s functioned in the same way; however, in later centuries, their functions diverged. While the *emīn* was a government appointee, the *mültezim* turned into a "contractor" who acted on behalf of the state.

29. Özer Ergenç has suggested an approach to the study of *muqāta'a* that empha-

sizes its administrative aspect and provides details on its place in the production process (Özer Ergenç, "The Sphere of *Muqata'a*: A Particular Dimension of Ottoman Spatial Organization and Control" [Paper delivered at the *İnalcık Conference*, Harvard University, Spring 2004]). I thank the author for providing me with a copy of his presentation.

30. BCR A-8/913, 25 Cumāde'l-evvel 896, April 5, 1491.

31. BCR A-4/1089 (Ali b. Abdullah); BCR A-4/2331 (Karagöz b. Abdullah); BCR A-8/1370 (İlyas b. Abdullah).

32. BCR A-8/2245 (Arab Oğlu Azadlusı Karagöz b. Abdullah); BCR A-4/1840 (Halil b. Aziz ve Karagöz); BCR A-4/1841 (Ali ve Karagöz); BCR A-8/1340 (Babamgeldi/güldi Mehmed); BCR A-8/1346 (Bekir Yusufi Elvan ve Hüseyin); BCR A-8/3569 (Emek ve Guri ve Süleyman).

33. For Balıkbazarı see BCR A-4/6121, and BCR A-8/3628; for Gallebazarı, BCR A-4/6121, and BCR A-8/3484; for Kanber, BCR A-4/6121 and BCR A-8/3628; for Tahtakale see BCR A-4/6121, and BCR A-8/4023.

34. BCR A-8/1314, 29 Cumāde'l-ākhire 896/May 9, 1491: "Brūsa'da Khassa Kharc Emīni olan Sadreddin b. Hüdadad şer'iyat mahfelinde ikrār idüb eyitdi ki: bozakhāneler kıstından 'āmil Salih b. Yusuf tahvīlinden emīn Seydi Ahmed b. Resul elinden ... yiğrmiikibiñ altıyüz akça alub kabz eyledim khassa kharca sarf itmek içün didi ŞH: mūsāb. Hasan; ve Hızır b. Abdullah; ve Dolı Mustafa b. Mehmed; ve kātib el-hurūf Mehmed." There were various other uses for *bozakhāne* income that accrued to the Ottoman government. It could also be granted to different social agents such as sheikhs.

35. BCR A-8/2982. All of these reductions were summed up in 1492 in a single document.

36. BCR A-8/3584, p. 261, 20 Muharrem 897/Nov 23, 1491.

37. BCR A-8/3628, p. 263.

38. Öcalan, "Bozahaneler," p. 118.

39. Kamil Kepecioğlu, *Bursa Kütüğü,* manuscript in the Library of Manuscripts and Old Publications: Bursa Yazma ve Eski Basma Eserler Kütüphanesi, Genel Kit. Nu. 4519, vol. I, 288, cited by Öcalan, "Bozahaneler," p. 118.

40. BCR A-8/6537, 22 Ramazan 897/July 18, 1492.

41. BCR A-8/ 6540, H. 897, 22 Ramazan 897/July 18, 1492.

42. Halil İnalcık, "Capital Formation in the Ottoman Empire," *Journal of Economic History,* 29, no. 1 (1969): pp. 97–140.

43. Fikret Yılmaz, "Boş Vaktiniz Var Mı? Veya 16. Yüzyılda Anadolu'da Şarap, Eğlence ve Suç," *Tarih ve Toplum: Yeni Yaklaşımlar* 1/241 (2005): p. 13.

44. Yılmaz, "Boş Vaktiniz Var Mı?" p. 11.

45. Yılmaz, "Boş Vaktiniz Var Mı?" p. 15.

46. Yılmaz, " Boş Vaktiniz Var Mı?" p. 24.

47. Yılmaz, " Boş Vaktiniz Var Mı?" pp. 27–28.

48. Laufer, "On the Possible Oriental Origin," p. 58.

49. J. L. Burckhardt, *Travels in Nubia* 2nd ed. (London: J. Murray, 1822), p. 201, cited by Laufer, "On the Possible Oriental Origin," pp. 56–57.

50. *The Message of the Qur'an*, translated and explained by Muhammad Asad (Gibraltar: Dar al-Andalus, 1997), p. 48.

51. *Message of the Qur'an,* pp. 111–12.

52. *Message of the Qur'an,* p. 162.

53. Ibn al-Ukhuwwa *Ma'ālim al-Qurba*, p. 84, and Yahyā b. Umar, p. 86, cited by Yaron Klein, "Between Public and Private. An Examination of Hisba Literature," *Harvard Middle Eastern and Islamic Review* 7 (2006): pp. 41–62.

54. Yılmaz, "Boş Vaktiniz Var Mı?" p. 46.

55. Kepecioğlu, *Bursa Kütüğü*, vol. I, p. 275, cited by Öcalan, "Bozahaneler," p. 120.

56. BCR B43, 77a, in Öcalan, "Bozahaneler," p. 120.

57. Kepecioğlu, *Bursa Kütüğü*, vol. I, 244, cited by Öcalan, "Bozahaneler," p. 121.

58. *Biz boza sarhoşundan dışarıya çıkamaz olduk; şehrimizi müfsitler kapladı.* (BCR B37, 34b, cited by Öcalan, "Bozahaneler," p. 120).

59. Evliya Çelebi, *Narrative of Travels in Europe, Asia and Africa, in the Seventeenth Century*, transl. Joseph von Hammer (London: Printed for the Oriental Translation Fund of Great Britain and Ireland, 1846–50), p. 13.

60. Evliya Çelebi, *Evliya Çelebi Seyahatnamesi*, ed. Yücel Dağlı and Seyit Ali, 4 vols. (Istanbul: Yapı Kredi Yayınları, 2001).

61. Eunjeong Yi, *Guild Dynamics in Seventeenth-Century Istanbul: Fluidity and Leverage* (Leiden and Boston: Brill, 2004), p. 109.

62. In this context, liver kebab resembles today's *meze*s, which are dishes similar to hors d'oeuvres served in small portions, much like Spanish *tapas*, as accompaniments to drinks in *meyhanes*.

Blending In and Separating Out: Sixteenth-Century Anatolian Armenian Food and Feasts

RACHEL GOSHGARIAN

In the mid-sixteenth century, a celibate Armenian priest named Xač'atur, most likely residing in the eastern Anatolian region of the Ottoman Empire, composed a text that reads: "If we didn't eat the meat of the pig, then we wouldn't be Christian."[1] The title of Xač'atur's text is "The Story of the Pig" (*Patmut'iwn Xozin*) and its discovery a few years ago in the Mesrop Mašdoc' Manuscript repository in Yerevan encouraged subsequent study of contemporary works that suggests that sixteenth- and seventeenth-century Armenian voices contemplating food and its ingestion occasionally use this subject matter to distinguish the Armenian Christian identity from the Muslim identity of their neighbors. This particular Armenian author, living in the tumultuous Anatolia of the sixteenth century, suggests that eating pork reinforces his Christian identity—ostensibly because pork is a meat forbidden by both Judaism and Islam (Muslims call it *ḥarām*).

By the thirteenth century at the very latest, Armenian authors had absorbed the concepts of *ḥarām* and *ḥalāl* as meaning "inappropriate" or "shameful" and "acceptable" or "correct," respectively.[2] These terms continued to be used in Armenian literature throughout the late medieval and early modern periods, but as the basic meaning of the terms *ḥarām* and *ḥalāl* became a part of an Armenian moral framework, that framework became devoid of any link to the specifics of the Islamic culture whence the terms came.

As Robert Thomson has shown, although Armenians came into contact with Islam quite early on in the expansion of the religion out of the Arabian peninsula, it was not until the late fourteenth century when the theologian Grigor of Tatʻew (in modern-day Armenia) wrote his "Treatise against the Tačiks"[3] that any sort of detailed and informed discussion of the beliefs and rituals of Islam was attempted.[4] Armenian authors discussed Islam during the eight centuries prior to this, but that discussion was rooted primarily in an evaluation of the origins of the religion and in the life of Muḥammad. Even in the aftermath of the composition of Grigor's text, as Thomson has discussed, Armenian literature seems not to have developed a coherent and complete understanding of Islam.[5]

This treatise, composed as part of his *Girkʻ Harcʻmancʻ* (or, Book of Questions), approaches twelve subjects related to Islam. Two of the twelve sections attempt to identify (and condemn) Islamic notions and practices related to the ingestion (or prohibition) of food and drink. One of the subsections deals with describing and condemning "those who eat all animal meat without discerning the contaminated ones" (*zpiłc kendanis voč ǝntren ayl zamenayn anxtir uten*), and the second addresses "those who refrain from drinking wine as *ḥarām*" (*zginin haram ǝmpen*).[6] The text approaches Islam from a fairly well-informed standpoint. Still, as Dadoyan has shown, large portions of Grigor's treatise make incorrect assumptions about Islamic dogma and practice.[7]

Even if late medieval Armenian authors were not completely aware of the belief system associated with Islam, Armenian literature picked up a wide range of the vocabulary, imagery, and thematic construct of Islamic culture. James Russell has noted, "An interesting feature of Mediaeval Armenian poetry is the Christian content of poems whose metre or imagery are familiar to most Western readers only in an Islamic context."[8] Centuries of contact with Muslims clearly allowed Armenians an opportunity to observe the everyday practices of their neighbors who adhered to Islam. It also provided the sort of environment within which they absorbed some Islamic terms and even cultural themes and, where food was concerned, reacted to those practices.[9]

By the sixteenth century, most Armenians lived either within the boundaries of the Ottoman Empire or under Safavid Iranian rule. Much Armenian literature of the time period reflects Armenian reactions to the ongoing conflict between the Ottomans and the Safavids, and it is during this politically tumultuous time period that writing about everyday urban life becomes a popular literary genre amongst Armenians in the poetic form of the *hayrēn*.[10] At the same time, it would seem that Armenian authors living in the Ottoman Empire began to carve out a very Christianity-based, exclusive notion of self that attempted to create—or express—cultural and religious boundaries through the written word. Given that these two trends were occurring simultaneously, it is only natural that a religion-oriented identity was carved out in literature by way of descriptions of everyday life. Food, one of the most basic elements of the quotidian, was also used as a method of distinction and differentiation.

Contemporary literature clearly alludes to norms and practices shared by Armenians with their primarily Muslim neighbors.[11] Still, those Armenian authors who wrote about food placed lines around certain cultural practices, sometimes alluding to similarities or links between Armenians and Turks and sometime writing explicitly about the distinctions between Armenian Christians and their Muslim neighbors. In many instances, food became part of the Christian-based cultural construct used by some sixteenth-century Armenian authors in order to differentiate themselves from their Muslim neighbors. This paper suggests that the cuisine-focused aspect of this cultural construct was erected in the sixteenth century as Armenians struggled between close social proximity with their Turkish neighbors and what was perceived as the purposeful destruction of their Armenian (and Christian) heritage as Ottoman and Safavid empires waged war against one another in Anatolia.

Much of Armenian literature composed in the sixteenth and seventeenth centuries addresses the sufferings of the Armenian people. During this time period, Armenians found themselves populating an area that had become a series of changing borders between the Ottoman and Safavid empires. Armenian scriptoria and monastic schools remained active during this time period. In fact, many great Armenian authors were educated and composed significant works during the sixteenth century. Kevork Bardakjian has referred to the century as one of "transition and regrouping rather than one of gloom and doom, as is commonly held."[12] Most Armenian authors—poets and otherwise—were priests or were educated by them. The Church offered them education and, despite its fractured state in the sixteenth and seventeenth centuries (with nodes of power existing at Ałt'amar, Constantinople, Eǰmiacin, Gancasar, Sis [Kilikia], and Jerusalem), it continued to act as the backbone of the Armenian people, offering them both religious direction and fulfilling practical roles of political representation under Ottoman and Safavid rulers.[13] That many Armenian authors from this time period either were priests at the time that they composed their works—or at the very least had some sort of religious training—naturally colors some of the concerns of the literature and explains, in many cases, the religious undertones present in the texts of the time.[14] Still, the wide range of compositions and positions suggests that Armenian voices were both plentiful and varied, in spite of the uniformly religiously-oriented education that was made available to them.

Armenian lamentation literature of the time often hearkens back to better days and calls upon Armenian saints who have passed away, asking for their direction during these dark days. For example, the sixteenth-century author Siméon of Ap'aran titled one of his pieces the "Lamentation for the Throne of King Trdat" (or, *vołbank' i veray t'axt'in trdatay t'agaworin, zor asac'eal e siméon vardapeti*).[15] The title of this lamentation makes a clear reference to Armenian Christianity and suggests a sixteenth-century concern with the early Armenian Christian past. The text was composed in 1594 in Gaṙni (in central modern-day Armenia). In the text itself, the celibate priest Siméon calls on Mesrop Mašdoc' (the fourth-century priest and creator of the Armenian alphabet) and asks him to "speak to us in your gentle (Arm., *k'ałc'r*) voice, because the nation is deprived of its light."[16] Much of this lamentation literature insists upon the Christian identity of the Armenians. Yovhannēs of Muš, a sixteenth-century monk from the Daron (Muš) plain, composed his "Poem on the land of the Armenians" (*t'ał vasn hayoc' yerkri*) in 1553. The text offers scathing criticism of the Ottoman advances into eastern Anatolia in the sixteenth century and bemoans the suffering inflicted on the Armenians.

> Dead are all our kings, / our country's princes gone; / And we, without a shepherd, / are pretty to the wolf-like throng.... Villages, towns and cities are all in pain, / Cloisters and monasteries also bear the strain.... The whole land is enslaved by the cursed Suleyman, / Descended from the conquerors Omar and Osman; / Taking

the holy churches, / they turned them south, / And exchanged the Divine Liturgy (*padaṙag*) / for the *lailaya*.[17]

Like many of his contemporaries, this text by Yovhannēs of Muš suggests that many of the woes experienced by the Armenian people were processed within the mindset of the clergy (or the religiously educated) as events that took place against Christians and that inflicted suffering on the Armenian people first as a Christian people and second as an Armenian one. This sort of interpretation is also prevalent in those Armenian language texts that deal with food.

Writing about food in Armenian and discussing food as part of an Armenian, Christian identity was not a new phenomenon in the sixteenth century, although the sort of literature associated with food did change over time. Many sixteenth-century texts discuss food in the context of personal narrative and should, therefore, be considered as part of the trend toward writing about everyday urban life that developed during this time period. Earlier conversations about food in Armenian were generally regulatory in nature. The earliest known reference to the relationship between food and an Armenian, Christian identity as opposed to a Muslim one came in the twelfth century when David of Ganjak (in modern-day Azerbaijan) wrote a series of canonical statutes, *Kanonakan Xratkʻ* (Canonical Advice).[18] His work became absorbed into Mxitʻar Goš's late twelfth-century law code, a text that was used as the basis for many centuries of Armenian legal practice from Van to Poland. In David's canonical statutes, the mixed feelings of the author towards everyday relations with the Muslim "other" are quite clear. In fact, he explains:

One shall not eat bread handled by an infidel [*aylazg*] nor drink wine or water tasted by them. Priests shall not drink anything left over by them or which their hand has touched, and this shall not be used as a holy offering. If there be a large quantity, it shall be used outside, and if there is but a little, it shall be poured away. Likewise milk and whey [*tʻan*], these shall also be poured away. If they should take meat, cheese or oil, that which has been handled shall be cut out and the rest washed and eaten. One shall not eat anything given by them—bread, cheese, meat, vegetables, grapes, and wine—except for those [fruits] which are in shells [or rinds]: walnuts, pomegranates, and melons, etc., and those things which are used to heal the body, apart from theriaca and other filthy [*piłc*] drugs.[19]

While the first sentence of this particular section of the text is quite powerful, it seems clear that David's opinion regarding food that has been touched by Muslims is changeable and varies according to quantity. If a small portion of food has been "soiled" by Muslim contact, then it should be disposed of; however if that portion is large, then it should be saved and eaten or drunk outside of the Church. The author's unwillingness to waste large quantities of food and drink that has been touched by "infidels" indicates the priorities of the author: food first and faith second unless, however, the sacrifice of food is small, in which case faith comes first.[20]

This conservative, and yet changeable, attitude of this twelfth-century author might very well have continued to penetrate various late medieval and early modern Armenian authors. In fact, a seventeenth-century Armenian text places Turks sitting at a feast alongside Armenian priests and laymen near Van, suggesting that Armenians and their Muslim neighbors did sometimes place their feet under the same tables and break bread together, in spite of any Armenian regulation against doing so. Composed in the seventeenth century by Andrēas of Arc'ke (Adilcevaz) near Lake Van, this poem was written as a sort of blasphemous *šarakan* (Arm., sacred hymn).[21] While the poem was most likely sung, it is doubtful that it ever would have been performed in church. The refrain, repeated after every verse, reads: "Intercede to the great barrel, bountiful is its wine."[22] A festive drinking song, this poem is filled with Turkish and Persian loan words—particularly for food—and presents a colorful picture of what feasting might have been like in late sixteenth- or early seventeenth-century Van, a city that had changed hands between Ottomans and Safavids several times but was firmly under Ottoman rule by the time Andrēas wrote this hymn to feasting.

Not much is known about the poem's author, other than that he had had a religious education, was apparently from the Van region, and knew Turkish well enough to write an Anatolian version of the Andalusian *muwashshah* in which he alternates lines between Armenian and Turkish.[23] This same author's festive poem, entitled "A Hymn of a Tale, Told for

Those who Write Poetry and are Kind and Happy," begins with a "satirical play on the Armenian hymns of the dawn office"[24] and details the range of foods present at a feast and the flowers placed on the table. The author uses several Turkish and Persian terms for dishes (although not exclusively). For example, he uses the Armenian term for the dish *herisa* rather than the Turkish *keşkek*[25] and although he makes reference to *kebab* he also uses the Armenian term for grilled meat, *xorov*.

> Most beautiful set of all tables / Filled with freshly fried fish/ Look again, what is there: / *Halva*[26] , *Porak*[27] and *Paxlava*[28] / A *łapama*[29] made of lamb / And filled to the brim with spices / The beloved *herisa* / And respected *k'allapč'a*.[30]

Andrēas goes on to mention a wide range of different foods: *lahana* (Modern Turkish *lâhana*, cabbage), *yaprax k'ufta*[31], *łaburła*[32], *ałavni* (Arm., sparrow), *pldrčin* (Modern Turkish *bıldırcın,* sparrow) and lamb kebab but insists that:

> The king is the grilled meat (Arm., *xorovac*) / And it's also the most beautiful: / Deep red of various shades, / The crown and luster of our table.[33]

The poem indicates that priests and deacons were seated at a table eating their food and drinking *arał* (Arm., alcohol)[34] and were joined by a group of Turks who participated in the meal's festivities, singing songs and making music.

> The priests and the deacons, / When they meet at the table / The bells ring, /And they sing together poems and melodies. / The Turkish rabble joins in / And listening to the various drums / They make music together with the *kamanč'a*.[35]

With this poem, Andrēas suggests a certain degree of "blending in" between these Armenians and their Turkish neighbors. The Armenian author uses Turkish terms for foods and eventually describes both Armenians and Turks sitting around a table, eating, singing and even drinking

alcohol together. Still, the meal is capped off with a Christian blessing and
a trip to church, clearly excluding the non-Christians present and indicating
a desire by the text's author to insist upon the Christian identity of the
Armenians, thus separating them out from the Turks.

> May you enjoy yourselves with this great honor / O, great ones and
> lords! / Eat and drink and make merry: / That is enough, as you
> well know! / Take pleasure from the Creator / So much goodness
> from the Giver / Bless, Father, Our Father who Art in Heaven! /
> And let's all get up and go to Church.

The abruptness with which Andrēas suggests that the entire table "get
up and go to church" after having eaten, drunk, and made merry together
suggests almost a sudden realization on the part of the author that the group
had blended almost too well together. Suddenly, it is time for the Armenians
to separate themselves out again, asking for blessings from God, making
reference to the *Hayr Mer* (or, Our Father), and encouraging a quick trip to
the local church, perhaps to atone for the worldly sins realized at the table.

Still, the image of priests feasting at tables decorated with glorious
foods and flowing wine was not a foreign one in sixteenth-century Armenian literature. One of the most celebrated poems on wine, entitled "A Poem
Celebrating Vineyard, Grape and Wine," was composed by the author
Astuacatur about whom little is known other than that he seems to have
enjoyed his drink.[36] While no Muslims are a part of this feast, the author
links the drinking of wine to the Armenian Christian tradition. In the first
stanza, the author refers to wine as the "expiatory of sins" making clear
reference to the Eucharist of the Divine Liturgy.[37] Further on in the poem,
Astuacatur describes the harvest of the wine by the hands of the clergy:

> Your color is a deep violet, / Red ruby [*yaǧut*, Modern Turkish
> *yakut*], precious stone, ruby [Arm., *sudak*] / The married priests are
> your cup-beareres / They preach and give out the cups; / The dea-
> cons heard, / And rose singing psalms / They honored you with
> incense / Picking it and bringing it to Church; / And they honored
> you again / On the altar they set you down, / On the Holy Table of
> the liturgy / By the hand of the holy priest; / To the life of the cup

of comfort, / The expiatory of sins and forgiveness, / Benevolent Christ's / Glory, Honor and Happiness / Oh fill and give! / Oh fill and give! / The sweet, chaste wine![38]

While Armenian poetry featuring images of wine long pre-dates this poem, Astuacatur does not use wine to communicate a mystical experience. Quite the contrary, he describes in detail aspects of wine in the everyday life of an Armenian Christian and satirizes, on the one hand, the notion that wine is part of a religious experience while at the same time detailing various aspects of that experience.

A contemporary, Martiros Larasarc'i (Martiros of Karahisar, about whose life almost nothing is known) also wrote poems that feature wine and feasting.[39] One of these, a poem entitled *Tał Vasn Uraxut'iwn Mardkan* (A Poem Concerning the Happiness of Man) details types of food eaten (grilled chicken, duck, and sheep) that has all been prepared in order to celebrate the "nation of the Armenians" (*hayoc' azg*).[40] In fact, the refrain, "let me bring the good news to the nation of Armenians," suggests that the author is making wine into the "good news." This table, too, is decorated with flowers and neighbors are invited (*hiwrer bazum ew drac'nis*), although the author doesn't mention if they are Armenians or Turks.

Happily drink six cups with me, / For the love of God or Saint Sargis; / Six ten and six, you win one hundred times, / Let me bring the good news to the nation of Armenians.[41]

Minas T'oxat'ec'i (Minas of Tokat, b. 1510) was a scribe who copied, illuminated and repaired Armenian manuscripts. He was secretary at the Armenian Archdiocese at Hackatar Monastary and the registrar of the Armenian court register in Kipchak in Lvov during the tenure of Archbishop Grigor of Van. Poor Minas of T'okat, having fled Anatolia in the early sixteenth century, missed his homeland and longed for the foods of his childhood while he toiled in Lvov. The poet reveals that his poem, entitled, "Ode to Herisa," was composed on Friday, February 5, 1563, after receiving an invitation from Archbishop Grigor to join him in his home on *Parekentan* (Arm., Shrovetide or carnival) in the eating of *herisa*.[42]

Herisa is a dish that has long been dear to Armenian hearts. As Russell has shown, in the Armenian epic, *Daredevils of Sassoun* (*Sasna Crer*), which most likely crystallized around the eleventh century, the dish represents equality amongst men as David, hero of the third branch of the epic, steals *herisa* from a church on the feast day of the Assumption of Mary prior to the priest's blessing the stew in order to feed his fellow shepherds who are starving in the mountains.[43] *Herisa,* amongst Armenians living in the Ottoman Empire, was a dish traditionally prepared on church grounds as part of a "sacrifice" (*madał*) offered to God. It was often prepared as part of the festival of Shrovetide, as is noted in this ode by Minas of Tokat, or as part of the sacrificial meal offered in remembrance of a deceased person. For Minas, the eating of *herisa* carried some spiritual value linked to Armenian Christianity and to his homeland. It is understandable that some might consider this ode to *herisa* a work of deep sarcasm as it so dearly discusses food and worldly pleasures in the context of the Armenian clergy (who were often times chided for their less-than-holy behaviors). However, the author of the poem—while a bit melodramatic in his praise for *herisa*— speaks enthusiastically of his love for food and links it to a nostalgia for the place of his birth.

> We have wound up in Poland's land, / And are bereft of everything. / We have become enslaved to the body / And have forgotten *herisa.* / I hope in the Lord of all / To have pity on us bounteously: / If he doesn't send us death too quickly / I'll return to our country.[44]

The poem underlines the fact that *herisa* is traditionally eaten just before the *mec pahk'* (great lent) during *parekentan* (carnival) or as a communal meal eaten in remembrance of the dead. The author ties *herisa* to Jerusalem, the center of Christianity and the primary place of pilgrimage for Armenian Christians.

> Hey, my dear *herisa*, / Everyone desires you / In Jerusalem, and everywhere, / There is no sacrifice without you.

More importantly for the local story is that Minas of Tokat distinguishes *herisa* from *keşkek,* although they are the same dish. In fact, he indicates that the Armenian *herisa* is better than the Turkish *keşkek*. While this might suggest that there was a slight difference between the two delicacies, it would seem that the author is claiming that the same dish is better when made by Christian Armenians than when it is made by Turkish-speaking Muslims.

> Hey, my praiseworthy *herisa*, / There is no one like you. / All men quiver before you, / And I am unworthy still more. / Hey, thou king *herisa*, / *Keşkek* is but a servant (Arm., *spasavor*) to you, / *Xorovun* (Arm., grilled meat) is your great warrior / And *pilaf* is your kinsman.[45]

Here Minas praises *herisa* to such an extent that he claims *keşkek* is "but a servant" to it. Given that in the Ottoman Empire, it was illegal for non-Muslims to engage Muslim servants, this one sentence in the poem might be considered a form of creative subversion. Minas also suggests that *herisa* is a temptress for Christian and Muslim religious men alike and intimates that the eating of *herisa* had similar distracting effects on Christians and Muslims who fantasized about eating *herisa* when they should have been dedicating themselves to prayer.

> A flock of the ranks of clergymen / When they hear of a dinner with you / Trade in their sleep, laughing mightily: / We will eat *herisa* aplenty! / When morning comes / They hasten to the church / But no prayers come to their minds, / Only, *When will the* herisa *come?* / All the ecclesiastical ranks of doctors / And the brother monks ascetic / When they see *herisa* / All commit apostasy. / All the Mohammedans / Drop their *pilaf* and *zardan*[46] / Their *boureks* [Modern Turkish, *böreks*] and their *baklava* / And come and eat *herisa*.[47]

Here, the author suggests that the promise of the ingestion of *herisa* has the effect of encouraging apostasy from amongst both Armenian Christians and Turkish Muslims. If the *herisa* encourages apostasy from amongst Armenians, however, it is at least inspired by what the author attempts to show is an Armenian cultural entity, making the apostasy seem less significant than a Muslim forgetting everything from his call to prayer, to his Holy Quran, and to his ablutions because of *herisa*. This very point is driven home by the author himself who suggests that *herisa* was actually created by Gregory the Illuminator, the saint who converted the Armenian King Trdat to Christianity in the early fourth century.

> Amongst foods you are praised: / The Illuminator invented you, / Made you and established you / And prepared you as a food for us.[48]

Minas insists upon the inherent link between *herisa* and Armenian Christianity. If the dish was, in fact, invented by St. Gregory the Illuminator as a food specifically for Armenian Christians, then it becomes clear that the author considers *herisa* a part of a cultural and religious framework linked to the very beginnings of Armenian Christianity.

While well-known Armenian authors like Minas of Tokat composed texts that insisted upon the superiority of the Christian identity of certain foods, lesser-known contemporaries wrote similar pieces. One of these such authors was a celibate priest known as Xač'atur. His above-mentioned "Story of the Pig" is part of a manuscript that contains the poetry of the twelfth-century Saint Nersēs Šnorhali, a reproduction of the thirteenth-century statute and canons of an Armenian *akhī*-like brotherhood by Yovhannēs Erznkac'i (of Erzincan), a series of advice, or wisdom, literature texts, and a reproduction of Grigor of Tat'ew's fourteenth-century "Treatise against the Tačiks." The manuscript seems to generally address what would appear to be many of the concerns of both clergymen and lay people in the mid-sixteenth century with regard to dealing with the Muslim "Other." The manuscript can be perceived as: an attempt to re-attach average Armenian-speakers with Armenian Christianity through the lyric poetry of St. Nersēs Šnorhali; an encouragement to create Armenian urban organizations as alternatives to the rapidly growing Ottoman guild system via the duplication of the canon of the brotherhood of Erznk'a (Erzincan); and also as an enthusiastic opposition to Islam via the "Treatise Against the Tačiks." Xač'atur's "Story of the Pig" is composed using a structure that more closely approximates colloquial Armenian than it does the classical language, suggesting that the author was not very well educated or that the author was, in fact, writing for an audience of the common people and not (uniquely) for the clergy. The author exhibits a real understanding of various illnesses and the concoctions traditionally made to heal them.

To the best of our knowledge, the text is unique and has not been reproduced anywhere else. Whether or not it is representative of a larger school of thought is not clear. Still, its existence shows that some Armenian authors were concerned with ensuring that Armenians were, indeed, different from their Muslim neighbors and insistent upon the fact that this could be demonstrated through food culture. The work is called a "story" (*patmut'iwn*) but it could easily be considered an ode to the pig. It begins:

Now, the pig is the cure for all pain. And in great quantities is useful for all of those who are of the Christian nation of God.... For tooth pain, it is a cure when placed on the tooth with smooth paper. And when ground with sugar it is a cure for eyes that have gone blind.... The meat of the arm, when cooked with wine and eaten, is a cure for the pains of disease associated with the gall bladder. And when mixed with garlic, then it is a good cure for anyone who suffers from a cold.... The throat of the pig is a cure for those who are sick with slander and slothfulness and when the meat of the pig is cooked it is a cure for hunger so much that even the kind Turk can be made well by it. Christians are supporters of the pig and eat it all the time.[49]

Xač'atur explains that the pig is useful for all of those who are Christians—the immediate assumption is, therefore, that it is not useful for non-Christians. While he links the pig to Christians, their illnesses, and their enjoyment, in some cases he intimates that pig meat is such a powerful remedy that even the hunger of the "kind Turk" can be quieted by it. In this text, the author first separates the Christian from the Muslim and then eventually blends the two together by explaining that the "kind Turk" might also benefit from the positive effects of eating pig meat.

In the second half of the text, the author justifies the eating of pork meat to Muslims. In fact, this section of the text is entitled, "a response to Muslims (*Tačiks*)." Xač'atur explains:

Now, we eat the pig for a number of reasons. Firstly, we eat the pig and reject the Jews and the heathens (Arm., *hedanos*). Secondly, according to God, it is holy. Third, it is useful in curing.

Fourth, if we didn't eat the meat of the pig, then we wouldn't be Christian. Now, you Muslims, you might not eat Pork, but you eat the meat of horses. And horse meat has no use, not in terms of curing or in terms of helping any illness. And it doesn't taste good to anyone and it is not written in any book that it should be eaten.[50]

Xač'atur's response places his concerns firmly within the framework of reaffirmation of his Armenian Christianness via cultural norms associated with food and explicitly discusses the differences between Armenian Christians and Muslims within the context of food. Taking the Jewish and Muslim law against ingesting pork and importing the reverse of the law into an Armenian Christian context, the author insists upon the fact that Armenians eat pork because they are Christian.

Armenian authors living in the eastern Anatolian provinces of the early modern Ottoman empire engaged with markers of cultural identity as expressed through the activities of daily life, including depictions of food and wine, feasts and celebrations. This trend in the literature developed as Armenian authors struggled to re-affirm their Christian identity as they witnessed a great destruction of their architectural heritage and observed first-hand religious and political transformations in Eastern Anatolia. The construct of Armenian identity that was developed in the writings of sixteenth-century Anatolian authors advocates a certain degree of blending in with their Muslim neighbors and at the same time encouraged a separating out from them. This two-sided policy seems to have been a reaction to the complexities of the religious, cultural, and political realities of the time. That even food and feasting were made a part of this attempt to control culturally the Armenians who were living in Anatolia indicates the central place of food as part of the culture of everyday life during this time period in the Ottoman Empire.

A Note about Transliteration

For Armenian, the Hübschmann-Meillet system of transliteration has been employed. For Arabic and Ottoman Turkish terms, the IJMES standard transliteration has been used. Most Turkish terms have been reproduced using modern Turkish orthography unless otherwise noted. In some instances, transliteration confusion may arise as the author has chosen to translate the Armenian reproduction of Arabic and Ottoman Turkish terms. Thus, throughout the text the term ḥarām *as a concept appears in Arabic transliteration. When quoted from an Armenian text, or discussed within an Armenian context, the Armenian transliteration is used and the term appears in the following manner:* haram.

Notes

1. Žołovacu, Xač'atur Abełay, Manuscript no. 1561 at Mesrob Mašdoc' Manuscript Repository (Yerevan, Armenia). The manuscript volume also includes: a copy of the *Kanonk' ew Sahmank'* (or, the Constitution for the [*akhī*-type, Armenian] Brotherhood of Erznk'a (Erzincan)) of Yovhannēs Erznkac'i, the sermons and advice literature of Yovhannēs Mandakuni, a fifth-century Armenian Catholicos and prolific author, as well as a chapter, "Treatise Against the Tačiks," from *Girk' harc'manc'* (or, Book of Questions) by the fourteenth-century author Grigor of Tat'ew.

2. While a formal study of these concepts and their penetration of the Armenian language has not yet been accomplished, it is quite clear that these two words were used frequently as early as the thirteenth century along with a slew of Arabic, Persian, and Turkish terms. In A. S. Manukyan's collection of thirteenth-century inscriptions, *Hayeren Jeṙagreri hišatakaranner JG daṙ,* (Yerevan: Armenian Academy of Sciences, 1984), the two terms appear repeatedly. In another work, *Colophons of Armenian Manuscripts*, ed. Avedis K. Sanjian (Cambridge, MA: Harvard University Press, 1969), these terms also appear in thirteenth- and fourteenth-century texts from various regions. Sanjian, p. 448, explains the meanings of the terms in the following manner: *ḥalāl* is "honestly earned," and *ḥarām* is used as "unlawful." In works of most thirteenth-century authors, including Yovhannēs Erznkac'i and Kostandin Erznkac'i, these terms and others not just from Arabic and Persian but also linked to Islamic practice are used frequently in an Armenian context. In fact in the thirteenth-century law code of Smbat Sparapet (the Cilician military leader and elder brother of King Het'um I), the term "*haram*" is used to mean unclean or forbidden. Section 175 of the code is titled, "For those who eat *haram* foods" (*vasn vor zumek irk haram uti*) (Smpat Sparapet, *Datastanagirk'*, ed. A. Galstyan [Yerevan: Armenian National Press, 1961], p. 150). Andrzej Piscowicz has considered the use of Arabic and Persian words in Middle Armenian in "How did New Persian and Arabic Words Penetrate the Middle

Armenian Vocabulary? Remarks on the Material of Kostandin Erznkaci'is Poetry," in *New Approaches to Medieval Armenian Language and Literature,* ed. J. J. S. Weitenberg (Amsterdam: Rodopi, 1995), pp. 95–109.

3. The term *"tačik"* entered Armenian meaning "fast" and was originally used to describe a horse or camel. After Armenians came into contact with Islam, the term *tač'ik* was commonly used to refer to Muslims. In the aftermath of the Seljuk arrival in Anatolia in the eleventh century, the verb *"tač'kac'nel"* appears, meaning "to become Muslim" (H. Ajaryan, *Hayeren Armatakan Bařaran* [Etymological Dictionary of Armenian] [Yerevan: Yerevan State Press, 1979, vol. 4, p. 365). Armenians living in the Ottoman Empire used the term to mean "Turk" (S. Malxaseanc', *Hayeren Bac'atrakan Bařaran* [Armenian Descriptive Dictionary] [Yerevan: Gos. Izdvo. Armianskoi SSR, 1945], vol. 4, p. 369).

4. Robert Thomson, "Muhammad and the Origin of Islam in the Armenian Literary Tradition," *Armenian Studies in Memoriam Haig Berberian,* ed. Dickran Kouymjian (Lisbon: Calouste Gulbenkian Foundation, 1986), p. 829.

5. Thomson, "Muhammad," p. 858.

6. Grigor Tat'ewac'i, *Girk' Harc'manc'* (Constantinople: [Astowacatowr Kostandnowpolsec'i], 1729), p. 51.

7. Seta Dadoyan, "Grigor of Tatev: Treatise against the Tajiks [sic.]," *Islam and Christian-Muslim Relations* 7, no. 2 (1996): p. 201. Dadoyan suggests that this is because Grigor bases his argument on the practices of a small sect of newly-converted Muslims with whom he came into contact.

8. James R. Russell, *Yovhannēs Tlkuranc'i and the Mediaeval Armenian Lyric Tradition* (Atlanta: Scholars Press, 1987), p. 6.

9. It is curious that while the term *ḥarām* entered Armenian vocabulary in the late medieval period, practices associated with the Islamic notion of *ḥarām* were not assimilated into Armenian culture. In fact, with regard to food and drink, most of the literature shows just the opposite: that what was *ḥarām* in Islamic culture (namely, wine and pork) was ingested heartily by Armenians, who even linked these practices to the Christian faith. With regard to using wine in poetry as a symbol of Christianity, late medieval Armenian poets describe drunkenness from wine as a means of communion with God. The thirteenth-century poet Kostandin Erznkac'i and the fourteenth-century author Yovhannēs T'lkuranc'i employed wine as a mystical actor in their poetry with great frequency. What seems to change in the sixteenth century is that poetry depicting wine drinking is less mystical and more jovial, featuring every day life scenarios while still remembering God and Armenianness.

10. Kevork Bardakjian, *A Reference Guide to Modern Armenian Literature* (Detroit: Wayne State University Press, 2001), p. 31. The *hayrēn* is a form of

Armenian poetry that deals specifically with daily life. It developed in earnest in the tenth century and became very popular amongst poets and bards composing works in the sixteenth century. See M. Abełyan, *Hin Gusanakan Żołovrtakan Erger* (Old Popular Minstrel Songs) (Yerevan: Armfani, 1931), and Asatur Mnac'akanyan, *Hayrenner* (Yerevan: Nairi, 1995). The poems can be divided into three groups: folk, minstrel-folk, and original. This form of poetry has a particular meter and versification: the poems consist of stanzas containing four fifteen-syllable lines. Each line contains two half-lines: the first is divided into three feet of two, three, and two syllables, and the second into three feet of three, two, and three syllables (*The Heritage of Armenian Literature*, ed. Agop J. Hacikyan et al. [Detroit: Wayne State University Press, 2005], vol. 2, pp. 1028–32).

11. In the fifteenth century, for example, the Armenian poet Yovhannēs T'lkuranc'i composed the story of Yovhannēs and Aša, in which an Armenian boy falls in love with a Muslim girl. The two meet in the village and their love story upsets all of the locals, as he is the son of a priest and she the daughter of the local *imām*. Their love is doomed until she converts to Christianity at the insistence of young Yovhannēs. See Russell, *Yovhannēs T'lkuranc'i*, pp. 104–17.

12. Bardakjian, *Modern Armenian Literature*, p. 31.

13. Kevork Bardakjian, "The Rise of the Armenian Patriarchate of Constantinople," in *Christians and Jews in the Ottoman Empire*, ed. Benjamin Braude and Bernard Lewis (New York: Holmes & Meier, 1982), vol. 1, pp. 89–97; and Vazken S. Ghougassian, *The Emergence of the Armenian Diocese of New Julfa in the Seventeenth Century* (Atlanta: Scholars Press, 1998).

14. Almost every author who wrote during this time period had some sort of religious education. For example, Zak'aria Gnuneac', a bishop who hailed from the region north of Lake Van, copied and illustrated a version of the Alexander Romance and wrote poetry dealing with the plight of migrant workers (the *laribs*) and love poems using the imagery of the rose and the nightingale; Karapet of Bitlis, who lived in the plains of Muš (Daron), was himself a celibate priest and wrote poetry and a lamentation on the invasions of the Safavid Shah Ismail; and Yovasap' Sebastac'i (of Sivas) was a married deacon who wrote on a variety of topics, including love, history, and the calendar.

15. King Trdat III was the first Armenian King to convert to Christianity in the beginning of the fourth century.

16. A. Madoyan and G. Ananian, eds., *Hayoc' hin ew mijnadarean banastełcut'ean Krestomatia* (Anthology of Ancient and Medieval Armenian Poetry) (Yerevan:Yerevan State University, 1979), pp. 528–38; translated in A. Hacikyan et al., *Heritage*, p. 775.

17. Madoyan and Ananian, *Medieval Armenian Poetry*, p. 501–2; Hacikyan et al., *Heritage*, pp. 746-49. The *lailaya* refers to the Arabic *lā ilaha illa Allāh* (Arab., there is no God but God), which is the first part of the Islamic declaration of faith and one line in the call to prayer.

18. The *Kanonakan Xratkʻ* of David was translated and edited by Charles Dowsett as *The Penitential of David of Ganjak* (Louvain: Secrétariat du Corpus SCO, 1961). Prior to Dowsett's translation, the text was studied by X. Samuēlean (*Hin hawatkʻ kam hetʻanosakan krōnkʻ hayocʻ* [Venice: San Lazzaro, 1910]), and by A. Aprahamyan (transl., ed., "Tawitʻ Alvka ordu kanonagirkʻ'" in *Ejmiacin* [Eĵmiacin 1952]: pp. 48–67, and *Ejmiacin* [Eĵmiacin 1953]: pp. 56–63), who recognized its importance in the development of Armenian law.

19. Dowsett, *Penitential*, p. 14. The original Armenian title for the section is "Concerning Muslims who Hold our Food" (Arm., *vasn aylazgoy zkerakur mer əmbřnē*) (S. Abrahamyan, "Tavit," p. 57).

20. Although much of David's work was "borrowed" by Mxitʻar Goš in the fashioning of his law code, this particular statute on food was not. In fact, Mxitʻar makes little mention of food, although he does define and condemn drunkenness and denounces feasting in monasteries. See Robert Thomson, ed., *The Lawcode [Datastanagirkʻ] of Mxitʻar Goš* (Atlanta: Rodopi, 2000). The code composed by Smpat Sparapet, which was fashioned for the most part after Mxitʻar's work, also includes a brief discussion of eating regulations and refers to certain foods as *harām*. See fn. 3 above.

21. James Russell, "The Praise of Porridge," in *Le Muséon* 116, nos. 1–2 (2003): p. 133, fn. 8. That Andrēas was able to copy the style of the Armenian sacred hymn in this satirical work clearly implies an intimate knowledge of church services and suggests that the author, similar to most of his contemporaries, most likely had a religious education.

22. Russell, "Praise of Porridge," pp. 129–72.

23. The *muwashshah* is a genre of poem that is strophic and that alternates between classical Arabic and the colloquial Arabic of al-Andalūs. Occasionally, such poems also include Hebrew and/or Spanish. Raymond Schiendlein, "Hebrew Poetry in Medieval Iberia," in *Convivencia: Jews, Muslims and Christians in Medieval Spain*, ed. Vivian B. Mann et al. (New York: G. Braziller in association with the Jewish Museum, 1992), p. 43, has suggested that the development of this genre of poetry in al-Andalūs attests to the "interaction of Arabic and local Hispanic cultural elements in a single literary genre and thus may be seen as embodying a kind of literary *convivencia*."

24. Russell, "Praise of Porridge," pp. 135–51; and H. Sahakyan, ed., *Uš Miǰnadari hay banastełcutʻyunə (XVI-XVII dd.)* (Late Medieval Armenian Poetry of the 16th–17th Centuries), 2 vols. (Yerevan: Armenia SSH GA , 1987), vol. 2, pp. 532–40.

25. *Herisa* and *keşkek* are respectively the Persian (and Armenian) and Turkish terms for a dish made of chicken and wheat that is boiled for several hours. "Keshkeg [sic, keşkek] is a very old dish that was served to pilgrims in the early Armenian monasteries. It is traditionally made with skinless whole-grain wheat that has been soaked in water overnight. The following day it is drained and combined in a cauldron with chicken or lamb and water. The mixture is then cooked and beaten for many hours until it attains the consistency of porridge" (Sona Uvezian, *The Cuisine of Armenia* [New York: Harper & Row, 1974], p. 143).

26. The term *halva* is used in both Armenian and Modern Turkish (helva) to refer to many dense, sweet confections that are usually tahini-based, but can also be flour- or semolina-based.

27. Modern Turkish, *börek* is a baked or fried pastry usually filled with cheese or meat.

28. *Baklava* is a sweet made of layers of dough filled with chopped nuts and sweetened with syrup or honey.

29. A Turkish term used frequently by Armenians, *lapama* (Modern Turkish *kapama*) generally describes a one-pot stew. In modern Armenia, the term refers to a specific stew that is baked inside a pumpkin.

30. *K'allapača* (Modern Turkish *kele paça*) was a Persian term that was imported into Armenian and Turkish and used to describe the garlicky soup made of the feet and heads of sheep. Sahakyan, *Late Medieval Armenian Poetry*, vol. 2, pp. 532–40.

31. Modern Turkish *yaprak köfte*, a dish of grape leaves stuffed with ground meat and cheese.

32. Modern Turkish *kaburga*, a roast of stuffed lamb breast.

33. Sahakyan, *Late Medieval Armenian Poetry*, vol. 2, pp. 532–40.

34. The type of alcohol this generally refers to is the non-sweet anise-flavored spirit known as *'rāq* in Arabic, *rāqī* in Ottoman Turkish and *rakı* in modern Turkish. In Armenian this term can also be used in reference to vodka.

35. The *kamanča* (Trk., *kemençe*) is a stringed instrument played with a bow.

36. Bardakjian, *Modern Armenian Literature*, pp. 296. "Author known for his only published poem: *yayn aṙajin žamanakin* [during that first time]."

37. Sahakyan, *Late Medieval Armenian Poetry*, vol. 1, pp. 71–78.

38. Sahakyan, *Late Medieval Armenian Poetry*, vol. 1, pp 71–78.

39. Bardakjian, *Modern Armenian Literature*, p. 414. "No biographical details are known about this author." His poems, many of which deal with feasts and festivities, have been published since the nineteenth century. Familiar with

several languages, at least one of his poems, *Tal č'ors lezuē laračarac'i martirosē asac'eal (*A Poem in Four Languages Said by Martiros of Karahisar*)* is composed in four languages: Armenian, Greek, Persian and Turkish. Sahakyan, *Late Medieval Armenian Poetry*, pp. 177–78.

40. Sahakyan, *Late Medieval Armenian Poetry*, vol. 2, pp. 145–50.

41. Sahakyan, *Late Medieval Armenian Poetry,* vol. 2, p. 147.

42. This particular text has been beautifully edited, translated, and studied by James Russell in a 2003 article published in *Le Muséon* using two original texts, the first from Fr. N. Akinean, ed., *Hing Panduxt Talasac'ner* (Five Migrant Poets) (Vienna: Mkhitarean Press, 1921), pp. 169–72, and "Govut'iwn i veray herisayi" (The Praise of Herisa) in *Sion* (Jerusalem: Armenian Patriarchate of Jerusalem, 1874), vol. 1, pp. 132–35. All translations of Minas' ode are Russell's.

43. Russell, "Praise of Porridge," pp. 130–32; *Sasunc'i Tawit',* ed. Manuk Abelyan (Yerevan: Armenian KHSH State, 1961), pp. 174–75; and Leon Surmelian, transl., *Daredevils of Sassoun* (Denver: A. Swallow, 1964), pp. 128–29.

44. Russell, "Praise of Porridge," pp. 138, 144–45.

45. Russell, "Praise of Porridge," pp. 138, 145.

46. Pers., boiled rice covered with saffron and sweetened; modern Turkish, *zerde pilavı.*

47. Russell, "Praise of Porridge," pp. 141, 149–50. The last stanza in the *Sion* version reads: "Their imams leave their table, / Likewise their *davat* (Trk., *davet*) and *Kuran* / Forgetting even the *abdast* (Trk., *ābdāst*) / When they hear of *herisa.*" Ottoman Turkish sing. d'vet, pl. d'vāt, meaning invitation, request, or summons. Given the context, one can assume that this is meant in a religious context, as in the call to prayer. *Ābdāst* (modern Turkish, *aptes*) denotes abolution.

48. Russell, "Praise of Porridge," pp. 141, 150.

49. 46 Xač'atur, *Patmut'iwn Xozi,* ff. 254 a, 254 b.

50. Xač'atur, *Patmut'iwn Xozi,* ff. 254 a, 254 b.

The "Michelin Guide" to
Public Kitchens in the
Ottoman Empire*

AMY SINGER

Tired travelers will welcome this opportunity to step into a calm,
wide courtyard away from the bustle and noise of the City. Located
in the heart of the main market district on a hill high enough to
catch the Bosphorus breezes in summer, this magnificent imaret
greets its guests with a reviving snack of honey and bread to tide
them over until the next meal is served. To the discerning man of
standing, a *sofra* (dining table)[1] is set at which he may dine with a
few men of equal caliber, enjoying satisfying stews and delightful
sweets.

If Ottoman culture had possessed the contemporary habit of reviewing and
advertising its public kitchens and guest houses, the above passage might
well have been penned to describe the imaret of the Süleymaniye complex
in Istanbul (Figure 1). Ottoman imarets have often been referred to as soup
kitchens. This is partly because the main item on most of their menus was
soup. However, it is also due to the fact that the English label "soup
kitchen" evokes a beneficent institution for feeding the poor, which is what

* I would like to extend my thanks to my co-authors, for their comments on early versions
of this work, as well as to Cemal Kafadar and Bill Blair, for their addition queries and
reflections. This research was supported by the Israel Science Foundation, grant #657/07.

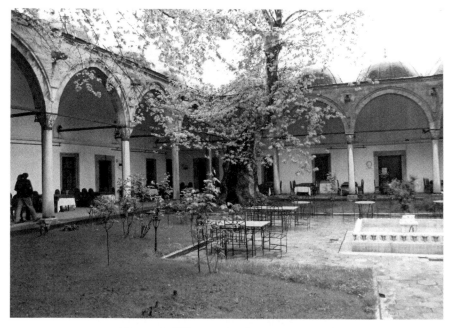

Figure 1. Süleymaniye imaret courtyard

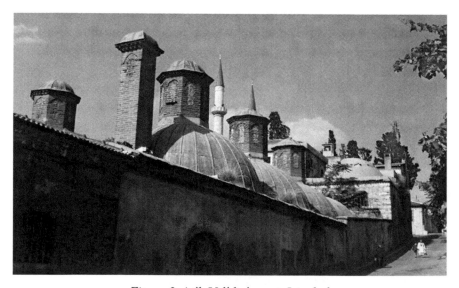

Figure 2. Atik Valide imaret, Istanbul

some foreign observers and many historians of the Ottoman empire have assumed the imarets to be. It seems, however, that not all or even most of the people who ate in Ottoman public kitchens were impoverished. In fact, although the kitchens usually did serve soup, local indigents were not usually the largest group of diners. Rather, the kitchens, founded throughout Anatolia and the Balkans and in some parts of the Arabic-speaking provinces as well, served a wide range of people, including imperial officials, travelers of different kinds, scholars and students from local *medreses* (colleges), Sufis, the staffs of the mosque-complexes in which the kitchens were mostly located, and also some poor people (Figure 2).[2]

This article examines closely the menus of several kitchens founded between the fifteenth and seventeenth centuries to investigate what can be learned from studying the similarities and differences in the food served in one kitchen or another. All these kitchens were founded as parts of endowments (*evkaf*, sing. *vakıf*), and the recipes (or at least the lists of ingredients) for the dishes they served were often included in their foundation deeds (*vakfiyes*). Additional information comes from Ottoman documentary sources such as expenditure registers for individual kitchens, literary evidence, and the reports of Ottoman and foreign travelers, all of whom availed themselves of the hospitality of imarets. Collectively, these sources offer detailed descriptions of the meals themselves, including the dishes served daily and on holidays, as well as some information on the quantities of food served and the settings for eating meals.

The broader context of the present discussion is a wide-ranging project on imarets in the Ottoman Empire, which is framed by a series of questions about how the imarets fit into Ottoman society, culture, and economy. At the same time, this close investigation of imarets across the empire (space) and through several hundred years of Ottoman history (time) aims to provide a new perspective on the nature of the societies, cultures, and economies we collectively call Ottoman. Previously, not only were the imarets assumed to be soup kitchens for the poor but imarets received very little focused attention at all. In most complexes, it was the mosques and *medreses* that were the showpieces, with all other institutions playing a supporting role. Mosques and their minarets symbolize more obviously the Muslim identity of the founders and the beneficent religious impetus behind the founding of the complexes. "Pray and pay alms" is a phrase repeated

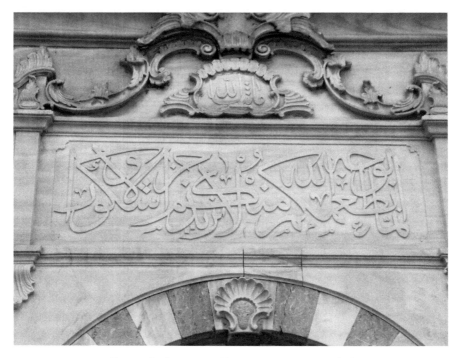

Figure 3. Gateway of imaret at Eyüp, Istanbul

in the Qur'an, recalling two of the five "pillars of Islam." The mosque stands for the first, and the entire complex might be seen as a sign of the second, though strictly speaking endowments are a form of voluntary philanthropy (*sadaka*) rather than obligatory almsgiving (*zekat*).[3] Yet the Qur'an does not lack for statements about food, such as the one found in Sura 76, verse 8–9, repeated in imaret *vakfiye*s and inscribed over the entrance of some imarets: "And they give from their food in spite of their love for it, to the poor, the orphan, and the captive [saying], 'We feed you for the sake of Allah alone; we desire from you no reward nor thanks'"[4] (Figure 3).

Although imarets may not have been the most expensive structures to build in any complex nor the most prestigious, they often seem to have consumed a larger share of annual endowment revenues than any other single institution in a complex. Not only did they require funds for maintenance and wages, like every other building and its staff, but also regular supplies of food, firewood, water, and cooking and serving equipment, in order to prepare and distribute meals. These included daily meals for the kitchen staff and all the other employees of the complex, as well as for the scholars and students in its schools, dervishes if there was a *zaviye* (Sufi convent) in the complex (or sometimes close by), other guests of varying rank, and some indigents.[5] Thus the historiographical status of imarets has perhaps not been commensurate with their historical importance. Instead, the focus on what were perceived to be the more noble elements of a complex of buildings, i.e., the mosques and *medrese*s, has been mirrored by the historiographical attention devoted to the most noble and notable *foods* of Ottoman culinary culture, that is, the dishes served in the imperial palaces.[6] And yet, ironically, it was the imarets which took the name of the whole complex as their own, as though they were the most important of its buildings. Osman Nuri Ergin observed early in the twentieth century that this was a popular synechdote, reflecting the concern of the populace for filling their bellies. Perhaps Ergin's interpretation hints at a change in imaret clientele from fifteenth and sixteenth centuries, when most were founded, to his era in the final years of the empire. During that difficult time, when refugees and the war wounded arrived in Istanbul in droves, the imarets were an obvious place to seek sustenance and support.[7]

The following discussion will first examine the basic dishes offered daily at several imarets before turning to savor the luxury fare served on special occasions and to diners of higher status and privilege. As Suraiya Faroqhi has noted, most of the evidence about Ottoman food culture before the nineteenth century sheds light on what people served at festival celebrations, on holidays, and to guests at home.[8] The festival accounts of imperial circumcisions and weddings and the descriptions of foreign ambassadors and travelers offer a guided tour, sometimes illustrated, of the feasts served at different Ottoman tables.[9] Providing a somewhat closer view of the usual meals of the majority of the population, sources like the *narh defteri* (book of market prices), published by Mubahat Kütükoğlu, offer a view of the wide spectrum of foodstuffs available in the markets of Istanbul.[10] The food prices listed there also help distinguish between common fare and delicacies. None of these sources, however, actually describes what "ordinary people" ate on a daily basis. For this, the imaret menus may offer a rare taste of everyday fare. The "reality check" for these meals prescribed in the *vakfiyes* can be found in the annual accounts registers (*muhasebe defterleri*) for the endowed complexes. These lists detail the foodstuffs purchased and stored in imaret pantries and storerooms and from them it is possible to confirm that the basic daily menu laid out in the *vakfiyes* was in fact what was served at the imarets in the relevant years.[11]

The prescribed meals described here reflect what the founders of the imarets imagined to be necessary and appropriate meals for the various people whom they intended that the imaret should serve. The comparison between several Ottoman imarets identifies the ways in which this Ottoman institution was standardized and to what extent it was reinterpreted from one place to another. Imaret menus were originally configured according to the vision and preferences of the founders, within the parameters of what was normal for public kitchens as well as what was conceived of as the luxury due to privilege and rank, the culinary markers that distinguished the less from the more privileged in Ottoman society (The unprivileged were those who were not even admitted to the imarets.). Thus, the study constructs a more nuanced appreciation of the culinary aspects of the imarets and sheds greater light on the practical and symbolic goals of the Ottomans in establishing and maintaining public kitchens over hundreds of years.

Thinking about the food served in imarets in a way comparable to how one might choose a place to eat today suggests new questions, such as whether the clients of imarets actually had options for obtaining their meals, and if so, what were the factors shaping their choices. A Sufi *tekke*, an imperial palace, the home of a wealthy person such as a vizier or other high-ranking Ottoman official, the home of the wealthiest person in a town quarter or village, or simply a better-off neighbor might each offer a free meal. In cities, there were also commercial establishments in the markets that sold cooked food; their representatives are described in Evliya Çelebi's famous list of the Istanbul guilds, together with the purveyors of all the different foodstuffs in the city. Illustrations of some of these foodsellers appear as well in the early eighteenth-century festival book of Levni.[12] Members of minority communities—Jews, Christians, foreigners, or even travelers from other regions of the Ottoman empire—could hope to find a meal at the tables of their co-religionists.

The historical version of the contemporary *Michelin Guide* presented below has been compiled in order to discuss the relevant data from different *vakfiye*s, with apologies to this famous French listing of fine restaurants. Each kitchen is presented and evaluated according to the following criteria.

- Name of imaret
- Location
- Description
- Prices
- Number of meals per day
- Meal hours
- Daily meals
- Additional foods
- Holiday meals
- Location of meals
- Who gets to eat

The rating system is based on the ladle, the kitchen implement generally used for serving soup.

 1 ladle = daily soups with bread

 2 ladles = daily soups with bread, special dishes on Fridays and some holidays

 3 ladles = daily soups with bread, special dishes on Fridays and holidays, some extras for important guests

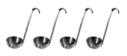 4 ladles = daily soups with bread, special dishes on Fridays and holidays, a separate menu for important guests, special service, and delicacies

Each of the "Michelin" entries includes: the name of the imaret, its location, a description that includes the other buildings in its complex, the price of meals, the number of meals served per day, meal hours, the menu of standard daily meals, any additions to these regular meals, the menu for holiday meals, the location of meal service, and who was eligible to eat. For the sake of comparison, we may note that today's *Michelin* restaurant guides judge the following features of a restaurant: the quality of the products, the mastery of flavor and cooking, the "personality" of the cuisine, the value for money, and the consistency between visits. It also lists items like phone, fax, website, wheelchair access, whether there is a garden/terrace, something about the wine list, and the dress code. Each restaurant is then rated "a very good restaurant in its category," "excellent cooking and worth a detour," or "exceptional cuisine and worth the journey."[13] Obviously, most of these categories are not relevant for the present discussion, but they do help to emphasize the extent of the difference between today's restaurants and the imarets, as well as the kinds of choices that were available then. Another difference worth noting is that the Michelin rating categories are based largely on the subjective, if professional, opinions of the reviewers, whereas the starting point for evaluating the imarets is the prescriptive conditions set out in the endowment deeds.

The imarets appear to share some common features, no matter what their size and location, nor how humble or grand the meals they served. Meals were free of charge. They were mostly served twice per day, morning and afternoon (*sabah ve akşam*). The morning meal was probably served after the early morning prayer (*fajr* or *güneş*), which takes place between dawn and two hours later. "Afternoon" referred to the time after the third prayer of the day (*'aşr* or *ikindi*), from mid-afternoon to sunset. Where stipulated, meals during Ramadan were served only once a day, after the sunset prayer (*maghrib* or *akşam*) that marked the end of the day's fast.[14]

Rating Imarets

The most common fare in the imarets, found virtually everywhere, was soup and bread. Specifically, in the morning the imarets served a rice soup made with clarified butter, onions, chickpeas, and salt, sometimes with the addition of parsley, cumin, lemon juice, or some other flavoring, in some places with the regular addition of meat; in the evening they served a wheat soup made again with clarified butter, onions, chickpeas, and salt, with the regular addition of meat in some places. In what is called here a one-ladle imaret, no other dishes were served. Such imarets may not have been very common, or perhaps they tended to be smaller, provincial establishments. Two such modest imarets (Figures 4–5) were founded between the years 1562–77 in the southern Syrian towns of Quneitra and Jenin, respectively, by Lala Mustafa Pasha (d. 1580), a former governor of Damascus, and his wife Fatma Sultan (d. 1577), grand-daughter of the last Mamluk Sultan, Qansuh al-Ghawri. Notably, they were founded in relatively small towns, and though the founders were a high Ottoman official and his well-born wife, neither of the two was a member of the ruling Ottoman dynasty. Their kitchens served only one meal per day—soup with meat and rice or wheat, and bread, and nothing special for people of status seems to have been on offer.[15] Rice and cracked wheat were the basic soups served most days of most weeks throughout the year at most imarets.

FIGURE 4

"Michelin entry" for Lala Mustafa Pasha imaret, Qunaytra

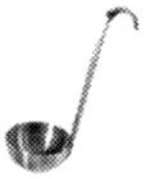

Location:	Qunaytira (Quneitra), on the road from Damascus to Nablus
Description:	*takiyya* (an Arabic word used for "imaret")*
Prices:	free
# meals per day:	one
Meal hours:	evening
Daily meals:	soup (one day rice, one day wheat), with one piece of meat, bread
Additional foods:	none
Holiday meals:	none
Location of meals:	not stated
Who gets to eat:	probably employees and some guests, one hundred bowls of soup

Takiyya is found in Arabic where Turkish would usually use *imaret*, however *takiyya* can also denote a Sufi lodge. This can be confusing, since Turkish would use the form *tekke*. The street in Jerusalem where the Haseki Sultan imaret is located is called 'Aqabat al-Takiyya.

FIGURE 5

"Michelin entry" for Fatma Hatun imaret, Jenin

Location:	Jenin, 26 kilometers north-east of Nablus
Description:	*takiyya*
Prices:	free
# meals per day:	one
Meal hours:	evening
Daily meals:	soup (one day rice, one day wheat) with one piece of meat, bread
Additional foods:	none
Holiday meals:	none
Location of meals:	not stated
Who gets to eat:	probably employees and some guests, twenty-five bowls of soup

Several practical problems prevent a good evaluation of the nutritional content of the dishes. While the specified quantity of each ingredient is known, it is not certain how much of each was actually used each day nor on average. This would have depended on the individual institution and the fluctuating competence and honesty of its employees. Many pots, bowls, and ladles remain from Ottoman times, but no work has been done to determine the average size of the soup pots (*kazan*), the ladles used to measure the portions, or the bowls in which the soup was served (Figure 6). Moreover, the lists of ingredients do not specify the quantity of water to be added to each soup pot. In one hadith, the Prophet recommends: "When you prepare a soup, add water to it, and have in mind your neighbors and then give them out of this with courtesy."[16] The Prophet's advice is impressive for its emphasis on generosity, but the attempt to serve all comers may end up diluting the soup to the point where it becomes neither tasty nor nourishing. In contrast, the size of the bread loaves is stipulated for some imarets: the standard loaf seems to have weighed one hundred dirhems before baking. However, setting all the unknowns aside for a moment, the ingredients do seem to provide a relatively beneficial meal that included basic proteins, carbohydrates, fats, fiber, and vitamins, despite the glaring absence of the fresh fruits and vegetables so highly valued in today's diet. Thus the simplest regular fare at imarets could have provided sufficient if minimal sustenance from a predictable alternation of rice and wheat soups with bread.

Even this simple fare of imarets, however, drew attention and admiring remarks from foreign travelers in the Ottoman empire. In his letters from the mid-sixteenth century, Ogier Ghiselin de Busbecq, ambassador in Constantinople from the Holy Roman Empire, described a meal he was served while staying in a *han* or caravansary. Very likely, the food there came from a neighboring imaret. "When dinner-time arrived, an attendant used to present

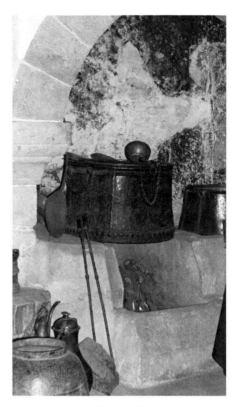

Figure 6.
kazan (cauldron), *kepçe* (ladle)

himself with an enormous wooden tray as large as a table, in the middle of which was a dish of barley-porridge with a piece of meat in it. Round the dish were rolls of bread and sometimes a piece of honeycomb."[17] Busbecq's contemporary, the Austrian traveler Salomon Schweigger, reported that: "Usually, a rice dish mixed with meat, a drink called *bosa* (boza) made from leavened semolina mixed with water, together with a loaf of bread are distributed to the one who asks."[18] The details of honeycomb and *boza* added by these two travelers (but not yet seen elsewhere) demonstrate how even simple fare might be enlivened with local variations.

In a two-ladle imaret, regular clients could count on having some weekly variety and the guests had clear privileges. The imaret of Haseki Sultan (Figure 7) in Jerusalem served everyone the same foods, marking

FIGURE 7

"Michelin entry" for Haseki Sultan imaret (Takiyyat Haseki Sultan), Jerusalem*

Location:	Jerusalem, west of the Haram, east of the Church of the Holy Sepulchre, south of the Via Dolorosa
Description:	mosque (*mescid*), fifty-five rooms, public building with imaret, bakery, refectory, storerooms, toilets, caravansaray, stable
Prices:	free
# meals per day:	two
Meal hours:	morning and afternoon; only evenings during Ramadan
Daily meals:	wheat soup in evening (cracked wheat, clarified butter, chickpeas, onions, salt, or cumin
	rice soup in morning (rice, clarified butter, chickpeas, onions, salt, plus sour labane and parsley (Arabic text) or seasonally zucchini/squash, *qushūr*, yogurt, verjuice, lemon juice, pepper (Turkish text)
	bread
Additional foods:	none
Holiday meals:	Friday: *zerde* rice (rice, clarified butter, honey, saffron); *dane* dish (*ruzz mufalfal*) (rice, mutton, clarified butter, chickpeas, onions, salt, pepper), bread
	Ramadan: *dane, zerde*, bread
	Aşure: four *kazans* of soup "*whose ingredients are well known*," bread
Location of meals:	refectory; Dajjani dervişes can eat in their *tekke*
Who gets to eat:	guests in the rooms = one ladle cooked food and one *fodula* bread (plus piece cooked meat on Friday)
	all staff members except manager, director and revenue collector (*vekil, mütevelli, cabi*) (thirty-four people) = one ladle cooked food and two *fodula* bread (plus piece cooked meat on Friday)
	four hundred of the poor and needy, weak and destitute, including dervishes = one ladle cooked food in a bowl per each two persons and one *fodula* per person (plus piece of cooked meat on Friday)
order of service:	imaret employees, caravansaray residents, the poor (who entered in separate groups): the poor among the learned, other poor people (apparently men), women

*St. H. Stephan, "An Endowment Deed of Khâsseki Sultân, Dated 24th May 1552," *Quarterly of the Department of Antiquities in Palestine* 10 (1944): pp. 170–94.

the distinction of rank and status by serving more food to those of higher standing. On Friday evenings, on Ramadan nights, and sometimes for the other festivals, a meat stew with rice and pepper called *dane* was served together with *zerde*, a honey- and saffron-flavored rice dish, and bread. These two dishes appeared together with the daily soups and bread over and over in the *vakfiye*s for imarets, such that they constituted a sign as familiar in the Ottoman cultural lexicon as a dome and minaret, an imperial *tuğra* (stylized signature), or an Iznik tile. *Dane* and *zerde* were on the tables at feasts, for example, on the *sofra*s spread for powerful and simple subjects alike at the imperial circumcision feast in 1539.[19] In fact, the dishes were so particularly Ottoman (in the sixteenth century), and not "Middle Eastern" or "Muslim," that the Arabic texts of *vakfiye*s for imarets in Syria included translations in order to explain what these dishes were.[20] Thus the imarets, where they were founded, may have been the first (and perhaps only) encounter of the non-elite local populations with Ottoman cuisine. On the other hand, for traveling Ottoman officials or merchants, the public kitchens may well have provided a welcome taste of home.

'*Aşure* pudding was another holiday dish that appeared in many imarets. Unlike *dane* and *zerde*, it was so familiar (and also had so many variations) that the *vakfiye* of the Jerusalem imaret simply listed it as "made with the well-known ingredients" without any further details. Curiously, however, even where '*aşure* pudding was not stipulated in imaret *vakfiye*s, it sometimes appeared in their accounting registers. One early nineteenth-century account from the Muradiye imaret in Edirne, similar to earlier accounts, recorded '*aşure* ingredients as including wheat, starch, honey, red and black raisins, black plums, pears, figs, walnuts, dates, almonds, beans, and chickpeas.[21]

Imarets can be further differentiated according to how expansively they celebrated holidays and how they treated their "guests," presumably higher-ranking diners than staff members or the poor. Partly on this basis, a tentative distinction can be made between a three-ladle and a four-ladle imaret. Another distinction between the two, although based on a very small sample, is that the four-ladle imarets are all located in Ottoman capital cities (here: Istanbul and Bursa), while the three-ladle imaret is located in Damascus.

In a three-ladle imaret, *dane* and *zerde* were served on all holidays,

FIGURE 8

"Michelin entry" for Süleymaniye imaret, Damascus

Location:	Damascus, in the Marja near the Baradā river, center of town today near University of Damascus
Description:	small mosque, twelve guest rooms, kitchen, bakery, storage rooms, two large dining halls; planned by Sinan, much larger than Salīmiyya; built on the site of Mamluk Qaṣr al-Ablaq, re-using materials from it
Prices:	free
# meals per day:	two
Meal hours:	morning and afternoon
Daily meals:	soup and bread, with one-half bowl of soup per person per meal, one loaf bread
Additional foods:	for guests: mornings – *dane* (*ruzz mufalfal*), sour gravy (*maraq al-ḥāmiḍ*), evenings *dane* (*ruzz mufalfal*) and sweet rice w/saffron (*zerde*), two loaves of bread each
	fodder for horses
	a bowl of food for the poor, added to each of the twenty-four guest tables
Holiday meals:	Friday nights and feast days: *dane* and *zerde*
Location of meals:	private rooms for guests; common poor served in the refectories
Who gets to eat:	ten people on two *sofras* in each of twelve rooms; eight hundred "common poor," but *faqīr 'ā'il* in the mornings, and then open to all in evenings

including "the two 'ids" of Şeker Bayramı/'Id al-Fitr and Kurban Bayramı/'Id al-Adha, as well as the minor festivals of Regaib, Berat, and Mevlid-i Nabi. Depending on the wealth of the endowment and its original stipulations, *dane* and *zerde* might be served on all the nights of Ramadan and not only on Şeker Bayramı. Sometimes *zerde* was replaced or accompanied by *zirbaç* or *zirba*, a pudding made with honey, saffron, red raisins, almonds, apricots, black plums, and starch.[22]

A three-ladle imaret offered some form of different meals to its more distinguished clients. At the Süleymaniye imaret in Damascus (Figure 8), the guests were regularly served *dane* in the mornings along with a sour

FIGURE 9

"Michelin entry" for Fatih imaret, Istanbul*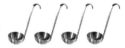

Location:	Istanbul, on the road between Edirne Kapı and the Grand Bazaar
Description:	mosque, *medreses, mekteb* (primary school), tombs, hospital, hospice, caravansaray, library, bath
Prices:	free
# meals per day:	two
Meal hours:	morning and afternoon, only evenings during Ramadan
Daily meals:	rice soup in morning with parsley, wheat soup evening, bread for both soups: mutton, onion, cumin, pepper, chickpeas, salt; in zucchini/squash season up to forty days of zucchini/squash and sour grape; in season, yogurt with chard
Additional foods:	guests: at most forty *sofras* for four people each
	on every *sofra: dane,* two *pare* meat stew, bread, *zerde* if necessary, sometimes sour stew with rice, black raisins, red raisins, figs, or black plums
	pickles of grapes, eggplants, and onions for guests and students
	for more important guests in the morning, sheep's trotters, pumpkin with honey, jam, cinnamon, cloves
Holiday meals:	Friday: morning wheat soup; evening *dane, zerde, zirbaç*
	ingredients: rice, oil, honey, red raisins, plums, almonds, figs, wheat starch, saffron, pepper, and the ingredients as listed for regular days
	Ramadan: one meal where the quantities for morning and evening are cooked together, *dane, zerde* and *zirbaç*
Location of meals:	refectory of imaret?
Who gets to eat:	(in order) the guests, the Fatih college scholars, students and staffs, the students from the nearby colleges and the dervishes, six hundred candidate students and their proctors, the staff of the imaret and the rest of the Fatih complex; the poor, when there is enough left over

*Fâtih Aşhânesi Tevzî'nâmesi, yayınlayan A. Süheyl Ünver (İstanbul: İstanbul Fethi Derneği Yayınları, 1953).

FIGURE 10

"Michelin entry" for Süleymaniye imaret, Istanbul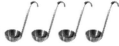

Location:	Istanbul, city center on the third hill, behind the Old Palace
Description:	mosque, *medreses*, *mekteb*, tombs, hospital, medical school, imaret, tabhane (hospice), bath
Prices:	free
# meals per day:	two
Meal hours:	morning and afternoon
Daily meals:	rice soup (with meat, and, seasonally, yogurt, spinach, sour grape, zucchini, carrot, parsley)
	wheat soup (with meat, salt, chickpeas, pepper, beans, cumin, gum mastic), bread
Additional foods:	honey for guests arriving; *dane, zerde, zirba*, sheep's trotters, honey
	for the *eşraf* (descendants of the Prophet): jam, pumpkin desert, grape pickles
Holiday meals:	Friday nights, Ramadan, Bayram, Regaib, Berat: *dane, zerde, zirba*
Location of meals:	refectory of imaret?
Who gets to eat:	staff; scholars; students; poor scholars and descendants of the Prophet, orphans studying in the mekteb, then the other indigents

FIGURE 11

"Michelin entry" for Atik Valide Sultan imaret, Istanbul*

Location:	Üsküdar, Istanbul (Asian shore), up on the hill high above the water
Description:	mosque, *medrese, mekteb, darülkurra, darülhadis*, imaret, storage rooms, *ribat/hankah*, hospital
Prices:	free
# meals per day:	two
Meal hours:	morning and afternoon; only evenings during Ramadan
Daily meals:	rice soup (parsley, meat, salt, chickpeas, onions)
	wheat soup (meat, salt, chickpeas, onions)
	bread**
	pickled grapes prepared with grape juice and mustard, pumpkins, sour grapes, thick yogurt

Additional foods: honey, given the moment someone arrives in the imaret (a traveler)

Holiday meals: Ramadan: *dane, zerde, zerba* (starch, dried apricots, dried plums, almonds, black & red raisins),*** *ekşiaş* (black raisins, fruit leather, mint, and cumin)****

Bayram mornings: "very nice and delicious dishes will be prepared"

Friday evening (= Thursday night) "a few different kinds of delicious dishes," including dane, zerde, ekşiaş

Other holidays: *dane, zerde, ekşiaş*

Mevlid: *dane* (meat, rice, oil, chickpeas, pepper, onions); *zerde* (rice, oil, honey, saffron, mastic) for "all the poor and needy who are waiting for it," and bread; sherbet (sugar, honey, *kandinebat* [a special sugar consumed at Mevlid], rose water)

aloe wood, incense

Location of meals: refectory, two hans, *tabhane* rooms for the lodging and feeding of visitors

Who gets to eat: in general—entitled guests, employees and the poor

specifically:

1. two full meals per day of one ladle of soup or some other stew, a piece of meat in the amount of fifty *dirhem* (silver coin) and a piece of bread in the amount of two hundred *dirhem*, for staff, scholars and students

2. fifteen full meals shall be given twice daily to the children who study the Holy Qur'an in the *mekteb*

3. the rest of the food shall be distributed to the needy, the poor and the residents [with no specified or guaranteed amount per person]

4. either *zerde* and *zirba* served together with *dane* on the *Berat* and *Regaip* nights and on holidays for the poor people living in the cells of the *hankah* and to the residents and to the coming travelers and to the poor among the town inhabitants, especially to poor elderly women [widows or women who never married] and other elderly pesons*****

* Vakfiye, VGM D.1766, as translated in Nina Cichocki (Ergin), "The Life Story of the Çemberlitaş Hamam: From Bath to Tourist Attraction" (Ph.D. diss., Minneapolis, 2005), Appendix 2.
** "Fodla: Bugünkü ramazan pideleri gibi ince, özsüz hamurdan, fazla mayalı, ekşice, lezzetli, kolay kopan bir ekmek. Daha ziyade imaretlerde pişerdi." (Sertoğlu, Osmanlı Tarih Luğatı, p. 114).
***The vakfiye gives ingredients as: starch, dried apricots, dried plums, almonds, and black and red raisins. Ünver says this was a kind of gelatinous desert made with cornstarch, sugar, raisins, and figs. It is also known as zirbaç. At Fatih imaret on Friday nights and Ramazan nights, it was served together with rice and zerde, for which see: Ünver, Fatih Devri Yemekleri, p. 28.
****In Fatih imaret, this was served to guests as they arrived at the guesthouse. Ingredients stipu-

lated included rice and [dried] black grapes, red grapes, figs, and plums, for which, see: Ünver, Fatih Devri Yemekleri, p. 8. In Atik Valide Sultan imaret, it seems to be made with black raisins, fruit leather, mint, and cumin. Sertoğlu, Osmanlı Tarih Luğatı, p. 14, defines ekşiaş as: "Akşıaşı: Eskiden imaretlerde pişen ve medrese talebeleriyle muhtaçlara ve uğrayan herkese verilen pirinç, kara üzüm, kırmızı üzüm, incir ve erik karışımı bir cins hoşaf."
*****The last line section seems to refer to the special dishes for this last list of people on the stipulated holidays.

FIGURE 12

"Michelin entry" for Bayezid II imaret, Edirne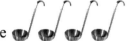

Location:	Edirne, on the banks of the Tunca river, north-west of the city center, south of the palace and the wrestling grounds
Description:	mosque, *medrese*, hospital, medical school, kitchen, bakery, hospice
Meal hours:	morning and afternoon; only evenings during Ramadan
Prices:	free
# meals per day:	two
Daily meals:	rice soup in the morning, wheat soup at night, bread
	clarified butter, onions, chickpeas for the soup
	[not clear if meat for everyone's soup or cooked separately for the guests]
Additional foods:	meat for guests daily, *paça* and fruit for breakfast
	honey and jams for guests
	fodder for their animals
Holiday meals:	Friday nights: *dane*, *zerde*, bread
	Ramadan: *dane*, *zerde*, bread, *helva baklava* Ideyn, Berat, Mevlid (and Aşure?): *baklava*
Location of meals:	refectory
Who gets to eat:	no clear details, but obviously the guests, and most likely all of the staff of the complex

* Vakfiye, VGM D.1766, as translated in Nina Cichocki (Ergin), "The Life Story of the Çemberlitaş Hamam: From Bath to Tourist Attraction" (Ph.D. diss., Minneapolis, 2005), Appendix 2.

---

gravy called *maraq al-ḥāmiḍ*. In the evenings they had *dane* again, along with *zerde* and two loaves of bread each. They also received fodder for their beasts. On each of the *sofra*s where they were served was placed "a bowl of the food destined for the poor," though what this was or how it was to be distributed remain unclear.

A four-ladle imaret such as the Fatih, Süleymaniye, and Atik Valide Sultan imarets in Istanbul or the imaret of Bayezid II in Edirne (Figures 9–12) served even more varied dishes on regular days and holidays and made sure that the guests ate their meals in comfortable surroundings. Beyond the basic rice and meat soups, these privileged diners received *dane* and *zerde* on a daily basis, or even tastier meat stews with dried fruits. Breakfasts would include *paça* (sheep's trotters) and perhaps some other treats. The imaret of the Atik Valide Sultan complex in Üsküdar included pickled grapes prepared with grape juice and mustard, pumpkin, sour grapes, and thick yogurt as part of the daily menu. In general, however, it seems that the special dishes were served only to short-term visitors. People who ate regularly at the imarets were served basic soups throughout the week with *dane* and *zerde* only on festival nights.

Results of the Survey

The simplest fare of the imarets may give us some insights into the diet of the laboring classes of the empire, but it would be unwise to assume that this is what they all ate regularly. For one thing, we know that rice, usually served in soup at least once a day in the imarets, and in the richer dishes on Friday nights and festivals, was something of a luxury in the sixteenth century, though it gradually became more common and more affordable, at least in larger Anatolian cities.[23] *Ferman*s (imperial orders) recorded in the *mühimme defter*s (registers of outgoing orders), for example, give us an idea of the effort expended to ensure a supply of rice to the imarets.[24] Moreover, those imarets that prepared their daily soups with meat were surely serving a meal beyond the means of most people, in cities and villages alike.[25] While the imaret soups strike us as minimal if satisfactory fare, they were probably still considered a substantial meal by many people. Having said this, however, we might turn to the Ottoman bureaucrat and historian Mustafa Ali, whose observations on imaret meals provide another kind of "reality check." Writing at the end of the sixteenth century, he said of imarets in Istanbul:

[S]ince their administrators (mütevellī) swallow their revenue, their food has ceased to be [apt to be] swallowed, their bread has become black as the earth and looks like a lump of dry clay, their soup has turned into dishwater, their rice and puddings into vomited matter, most of their stewed meat (yakhnī) is made of the meat of emaciated sheep that were slaughtered after having died. Things have come to such a pass that those who descend at their establishments [travelers] settle there only for residence. When the time comes for having a meal they wander off to Taḥtaqal'e. The *medrese* students who are assigned food there, on the other hand, come solely to meet with their colleagues; they pour their soup to the dogs, and they themselves stay hungry and withdraw after for a while having filled the air with the hullabaloo of the metal soup bowls.[26]

Mustafa Ali, having left us such a vile description of the Istanbul imarets, follows this with an utterly mouth-watering catalogue of the treats awaiting someone who visited one of the imarets built by Evrenos Bey in Rumeli in the fourteenth century.

Evrenos Beg has [left behind] . . . three flourishing soup-kitchens and first-class charitable establishments well-stocked with food. . . . twice a day four or five kinds of food are distributed freely to the travellers and when notables or high personages make halt there the amounts are doubled. Furthermore, during the meal each person receives a bowl of honey-*sherbet* and after the meal delicious fruits of various kind according to the season, and every night the abode of each notable is illuminated by a candle. The guests, not only *begs*, *sipāhīs*, and *za'ims*, are given a ration of fodder for horses and mounts. Visitors commanding respect are honored at the time of their departure with a box of sweet confection (*ghāzīler helvāsı*) as a nourishment of the soul. . . . These institutions are so efficient, the food offered to the travellers is so delicious and soul-nourishing as it has been mentioned and even more delicious and more pleasant than the food prepared by home-trained cooks. Their stewed meat is well-seasoned, their soup and hamburgers are plen-

tiful, and their noodles and noodle soup are of equal quality. Moreover, during the nights of the fast there are always on every table
a *baqlava* like the disk of the shining moon and sweeter than sugar,
and countless tasty delicacies of the sausage (*būmbār*) and *herīse*
(kind of meal pudding) type. As a matter of fact this humble [au-
thor] has repeatedly been a guest in these institutions and has found
its boundless delicacies even more than what we have said here.[27]

Mustafa Ali's seemingly exaggerated condemnation and praise of the
imarets nonetheless remind us that conditions in them could vary wildly
from one to the next, as well as from what their founders had originally
prescribed. Nonetheless, they offer a view into the terms used by a
contemporary in evaluating the imarets.

As is evident in many published sources and research works on
Ottoman culinary traditions, the meals concocted for people of standing
were progressively richer in terms of the numbers of ingredients and varieties of meats and fruits. Rice, wheat, and bread remained as the staple an-
chor of all these meals, and we should assume that there were many at least
minor deviations from the terms of the *vakfiye*s when composing meals for
the notables who arrived at an imaret, if only due to seasonal changes in
available produce at the markets and perhaps the whim of the cook or even
the guest. Unlike today's food aficianados, travelers in the Ottoman empire
were unlikely to "make a detour" or even a special journey in order to eat
in an imaret; indeed, research has not yet clarified whether potential clients
could seek out one imaret, or one particular source of food (i.e., private
home, Sufi *tekke*) over another, when faced with a choice. To date, most
sources present the perspective of the institutions and not the potential con-
sumers. Essentially, the imarets were located in such a way as to present
local customers and travelers alike with a convenient place to eat close to
where they had a bed for the night, mostly in towns but sometimes in the
countryside. Yet in some of these places, diners could look forward to a
meal that might have impressed even the authors of the *Guide Michelin*.

Notes

1. A wood or metal tray used as a dining table. Alternately, a *sofra* may refer to
   a leather or textile mat spread out, on which food is served.

2. For a general discussion of imarets, see: A. Singer, "Imarets," in *The Ottoman World*, ed. Christine Woodhead (London: Routledge, forthcoming).

3. On *zekat* and *sadaka*, see Amy Singer, *Charity in Islamic Societies* (Cambridge: Cambridge University Press, 2008), chapters 1 and 2.

4. This inscription is found over the gateway of the Eyüp imaret in Istanbul as well as over the doorway to the Süleymaniye imaret in Damascus, for which see: Astrid Meier, "For the Sake of God Alone? Food Distribution Policies, *Takiyya*s and Imarets in Early Ottoman Damascus," in *Feeding People, Feeding Power: Imarets in the Ottoman Empire*, ed. Nina Ergin, Christoph K. Neumann, and Amy Singer (İstanbul: Eren Yayınları, 2007), p. 121.

5. These details are discussed in Amy Singer, *Constructing Ottoman Beneficence: An Imperial Soup Kitchen in Jerusalem* (Albany: State University of New York Press, 2002), pp. 54–65, based primarily on the *vakfiye* texts of the Süleymaniye in Istanbul and the Haseki Sultan imaret in Jerusalem, for which see: Kemal Edib Kürkçüoğlu, *Süleymaniye Vakfiyesi* (Ankara: Resimli Posta Matbaası, 1962), and St. H. Stephan, "An Endowment Deed of Khâsseki Sultân, Dated 24th May 1552," *Quarterly of the Department of Antiquities in Palestine* 10 (1944): pp. 170–94.

6. Suraiya Faroqhi, "Introduction," in *The Illuminated Table, the Properous House: Food and Shelter in Ottoman Material Culture*, ed. Suraiya Faroqhi and Christoph K. Neumann (Wüzburg: Ergon-Verlag, 2003), pp. 23–24; see also Tülay Artan, "Aspects of the Ottoman Elite's Food Consumption: Looking for 'Staples,' 'Luxuries,' and 'Delicacies,' in a Changing Century," in *Consumption Studies and the History of the Ottoman Empire, 1550–1922: An Introduction*, ed. Donald Quataert (Albany: SUNY Press, 2000), pp. 107–200; Omer Lutfi Barkan, "Saray Mutfağının 894–895 (1489–1490) Yılına Âit Muhasebe Bilançosu," *İstanbul Üniversitesi İktisat Fakültesi Mecmuası* 23, no. 1–2 (Ekim–Şubat 1962–63): pp. 380–98; Hedda Reindl-Kiel, "The Chickens of Paradise: Official Meals in the Mid-Seventeenth-Century Ottoman Palace," in *The Illuminated Table*, ed. Faroqhi and Neumann, pp. 59–88; Zeynep Tarım Ertuğ, "The Ottoman Imperial Kitchens as Imarets," in *Feeding People, Feeding Power*, ed. Ergin, Neumann, Amy Singer, pp. 251–59; and Stephanos Yerasimos, *Sultan Sofraları: 15. ve 16. Yüzyılda Osmanlı Saray Mutfağı* (İstanbul: Yapı ve Kredi Yayınları, 2002).

7. Osman N. Ergin, *Türk Şehirlerinde İmâret Sistemi* (İstanbul: Cumhuriyet Matbaası, 1939), pp. 8–15.

8. See the section by Halil Inalcik on Ottoman kitchens, in D. Waines, H. Inalcık, and J. Burton-Page, "*Matbakh*," in *Encyclopaedia of Islam*, 2nd ed. (Leiden: Brill, 1960–2003), vol. 6, pp. 809–13, and Suraiya Faroqhi, *Subjects of the Sultan: Culture and Daily Life in the Ottoman Empire* (London: I.B. Tauris, 2000), p. 204.

9. For the experience of one ambassador, see the article by Joanita Vroom in this volume. Mouth-watering descriptions and some wonderful illustrations of these feasts can be found in the volumes written and illustrated to commemorate the events. Two of the most famous are the 1582 *Surname* and the *Surname of Levni* from the early eighteenth century, both found in manuscript in the Topkapı Palace Library in Istanbul. They were published, respectively, by Nurhan Atasoy, *1582 Surname-i Hümayun: An Imperial Celebration* (İstanbul: Koçbank, 1997), and Esin Atıl, *Levni and the Surname: The Story of an Eighteenth-Century Ottoman Festival* (Seattle: University of Washington Press, 2000). Other representative accounts of feasts include Semih Tezcan, *Bir Ziyafet Defteri* (İstanbul: Simurg Yayıncılık, 1998), and the letters of Lady Mary Wortley Montagu, *The Complete Letters of Lady Mary Wortley Montagu*, ed. Robert Halsband, 3 vols. (Oxford: Clarendon Press, 1966–67).

10. Mübahat Kütükoğlu, *Osmanlılarda Narh Müessesesi ve 1640 Tarihli Narh Defteri* (İstanbul: Enderun Kitabevi, 1983).

11. Several such accounts for imarets were published by Ömer Lutfi Barkan: "Fatih Câmi ve İmareti Tesîslerinin 1489–1490 Yıllarına âit Muhasebe Bilânçoları," *İstanbul Üniversitesi İktisat Fakültesi Mecmuası* 23, no. 1–2 (1962–63): pp. 297–341; "Edirne ve Civarındaki Bazı İmaret Tesislerinin Yıllık Muhasebe Bilançoları," *Belgeler* 1, no. 2 (1964): pp. 235–377; and "Süleymaniye Camii ve İmareti Tesislerine ait Yıllık Bir Muhasebe Bilânçosu 993–994 (1585–1586)," *Vakıflar Dergisi* 9 (1971): pp. 109–62.

12. See Evliya Çelebi, *Evliya Çelebi Seyahatnamesi*, 1. Kitap: *İstanbul*, prepared by Orhan Şaik Gökyay (Istanbul: Yapı Kredi Yayınları, 1996), pp. 227 ff.; Atıl, *Levni and the Surname*; and http://www.kanyak.com/surname-i-vehbi/images.html (accessed Feb. 26, 2010). For banquet images on the website, see: 22b–23a, 43b–44a, 58b–59a, 68b–69a, 85b–86a, and 122b–123a; for urban food supply and preparation images, see: 75b–76a, 77b–78a, and 107b–108a. Atil's book has slightly different numbering, and does not include all of the images listed here.

13. http://www.michelinguide.com/us/ratings.html (accessed 8 July 2009).

14. See A. Süheyl Ünver, *Fatih Devri Yemekleri* (İstanbul: İstanbul Üniversitesi Tıp Tarihi Enstitüsü, 1952), pp. 78–79. Ünver editorializes a fair amount about today's eating habits as compared with the more spartan ones of an earlier era and praises the two-meal day for contributing to better work habits, where meals provided a time for a break. He says that two meals per day was the norm throughout society. Thus, the imaret illustrates one aspect of the daily routine and rhythm.

15. Astrid Meier, "For the Sake of God Alone? Food Distribution Policies, *Takiyya*s and Imarets in Early Ottoman Damascus," in *Feeding People, Feeding Power*, ed. Ergin, Neumann, and Singer, pp. 136, 142.

16. Muslim ibn Ḥajjāj al-Qushayrī, *Sahih Muslim*, Book 032, "Al-birr wa'l-salat wa'l-adab," Chapter 40, Number 6358, http://www.usc.edu/dept/MSA/fundamentals/hadithsunnah/muslim/032.smt.html (accessed on March 27, 2007)

17. Ogier Ghiselin de Busbecq, *The Turkish Letters of Ogier Ghiselin de Busbecq, Imperial Ambassador at Constantinople 1554–1562*, trans. Edward Seymour Forster (Baton Rouge: Louisiana State University Press, 2005), p. 18.

18. Salomon Schweigger, *Sultanlar Kentine Yolculuk 1578–1581* (İstanbul: Kitap Yayınevi, 2004), p. 128. On *boza*, see the article by İklil O. Selçuk, "State Meets Society: A Study of *Bozakhāne* Affairs in Bursa," in this volume.

19. Semih Tezcan, *Bir Ziyafet Defteri* (İstanbul: Simurg Yayıncılık, 1998).

20. For example, *mā sammathu al-arwām yakhnī* (what the Rum call *yahne*) (*Kitāb Waqf al-Wazīr Lālā Muṣṭafá Bāshā wa-Yalīhi Kitāp Waqf Fāṭima Khātūn bint Muḥammad Bik ibn al-Sulṭān al-Malik al-Ashraf Qānṣawh al-Ghawrī*, waqafa ʿalá ṭabʿihimā Khalīl ibn Aḥmad Mardam [Dimashq: Maṭbaʿat al-ʿUmūmiyya, 1955], p. 221); *al-taʿām al-ḥulw al-maʿrūf bi-zarda* (the sweet dish known as *zerde*) (Muḥammad M. Arnāʾūṭ, *Muʿṭayāt ʿan Dimashq wa-Bilād al-Shām al-Janūbiyyah fī nihāyat al-qarn al-sādis ʿashar: Waqfiyyat Sinān Bāshā* [Dimashq: Dār al-Ḥaṣād, 1993], p. 160). These two examples are taken from Meier, "For the Sake of God Alone," 143, n. 125.

21. Başbakanlık Osmanlı Arşivi, D.HMH.21950 (1250 AH).

22. Kemal Edib Kürkçüoğlu, *Süleymaniye Vakfiyesi* (Ankara: Resimli Posta Matbaası, 1962), pp. 157 (Ottoman text), 43 (Turkish transliteration); "Zırva: Musavi ölçüde şeker, nişasta, kuru üzüm ve incirle pişirilen bir cins tatlı" (Midhat Sertoğlu, *Osmanlı Tarih Luğatı*, düzeltilmiş ve ilaveli 2. baskı [İstanbul: Enderun Kitabevi, 1986], p. 374).

23. Faroqhi, *Subjects of the Sultan*, pp. 206–7, writes that rice was something of a luxury but it is a standard item on imaret menus and listed as distributed to all diners.

24. Uriel Heyd, *Ottoman Documents on Palestine 1552–1615* (Oxford: Oxford University Press, 1960).

25. Faroqhi, *Subjects of the Sultan*, p. 207.

26. Mustafa Ali, *Muṣṭafá ʿĀlī's Counsel for Sultans of 1581*, ed., trans., and notes by Andreas Tietze, 2 vols (Vienna: Verlag der Österreichischen Akademie der Wissenschaften, 1979–82), vol. 2, p. 27.

27. Mustafa Ali, *Muṣṭafá ʿĀlī's Counsel for Sultans*, vol. 2, p. 28.

Ahmed I's Hunting Parties: Feasting in Adversity, Enhancing the Ordinary*

TÜLAY ARTAN

Certainly in medieval and also in early modern societies, many if not all ruling elites had their origins in warfare, which eventually configured them as warrior nobilities, or at least as the "military class" (*askerîs*) of Ottoman parlance. The ethos thereby created required the warrior lord to maintain his martial and chivalric identity in peacetime, too, through activities that resembled or approximated war. Apart from the knightly tournament in Europe, hunting was the closest substitute or surrogate, because like war, it demanded expense met without complaint. One had to be well-horsed and well-armed. Moreover, the hunter had to conceal fear and be vigorous, make do with a poor bed or no bed when necessary, rise early, tolerate both heat and cold, and suffer a lack of good food and drink.[1]

Of course, monarchs, princes and the upper classes hunted not only as part of a military training exercise, but also as part of their legacy—it was a birthright.[2] It became a rite of initiation; and it stood out as a prominent symbol and manifestation of power. Furthermore, beyond all the similarities between the hardships of war and of hunting, in the end there was venison only for the latter.

---

*My title takes off from: Nicola Fletcher, *Charlemagne's Tablecloth. A Piquant History of Feasting* (New York: Saint Martin's Press, 2005), p. 75.

93

In Europe, hunting deer and wild boar was strictly reserved for the aristocracy.[3] This opened up to an entire social context in which especially poetic references to the hunt assumed that the chase and the party were synonymous. All across Eurasia, hunting, eating, drinking, and making merry emerged as a common theme. In his comprehensive study on the subject, Thomas Allsen remarks that this is particularly true of the "core" area in which Sasanid and then Islamic art came to associate closely the notion of paradise, whether in this life or the next, with hunting and banqueting.[4] Persian kings, before and after Islam, provided hunting feasts, as did Mongolian khans, Hindu rajahs, Manchu emperors, and Romanov tsars in Russia.[5]

Ottoman Hunting and Banqueting

The Ottoman royal hunt (and the accompanying banquet) figures only vaguely in this picture.[6] Despite their wealth, primary sources have some problems. While the available narrative sources do record numbers of hunting expeditions, these are mostly in the nature of generic references which do not reflect either the actual practices or the related ceremonies in any detail. Likewise, miniatures depicting the Ottoman hunter-sultan, which emulate the constructs of the eleventh-century Persian epic, the *Shahname* of Firdausi, have mostly served as a strictly formal structure for exalting sovereignty. Furthermore, no hunting banquet appears to have been illustrated in the Ottoman versions of the book of kings.

Banqueting scenes, however, abound in Islamic miniatures, and these have been the subject of some debate. "The two motifs," argues Dorothy Shepherd, "banquet and hunt, when taken together correspond precisely to the late classical iconography of heroization. They represent the banquet and hunt in paradise."[7] She goes on to insist that the scenes of celestial hunting and banqueting are accompanied by those of death and funeral (designed, perhaps, as pairs), providing positive confirmation for "victory over death," celebrated with feasting and drinking, music and entertainment. "When the hunt—or more rarely some other equestrian activity—is added, it is only an adjunct, an embellishment, to the main subject and normally has no special iconographic features of its own." She argues that the courtly art of the Sasanians never existed and continues to claim that "this is apparently equally true of Islamic art": these princely themes were intended to represent or at least to remind one of the rewards of the *afterlife*.

This argument can be tackled on several levels. For the moment, suffice it to note that, very much like an obsolete canon of the history of Ottoman literature which insists that Ottoman poetry had nothing to do with human love and was only concerned with mystic, allegorical infatuation,[8] any purely symbolic description of Ottoman visuality solely by reference to a canon (Islamic or pre-Islamic) made up of repetitive and strictly rule-bound "medieval" formats denies the larger context of the historical processes through which paintings included in illustrated biographical histories were produced and, in so doing, limits our understanding of Ottoman culture.

Now if we go back to real life, we do know that several types of hunting were involved: hunting with prized birds of prey in the royal gardens of the capital; sedan or armchair hunting (*araba, oturak*) in the vicinity of the hunting lodges in Istanbul; the chase and the drive (battue: *sürgün, sürek*) in hunting parks that were mostly in the vicinity of Edirne or beyond. Hunting in the air required high-flying falcons and low-flying sparrow-hawks and goshawks. For the capture of both birds and small furry game, the battue involved a beating of woods and underbrush to drive game out toward hunters. For hunting with birds of prey, the sultan and his retinue moved from one royal garden to the other, mostly on the waterfront and also near springs of fresh water. This largely entailed sight-seeing, at ease and in luxury. When the Ottoman hunter-sultan participated in a large-scale chase or drive in person, he hunted only with bows and arrows.

with birds of prey was still a largely pleasurable princely habit. The chase or drive often turned into an extravagant show, incorporating aggressive fighting with jolly partying afterwards.

Celalzâde Mustafa Çelebi writes, for example, that Süleyman I wanted to clear his mind and go hunting in Beykoz and then in Yalova in 1533. The hunt was accompanied afterwards with music and feasting (*gülveş safâ-bahş ateşler yakub ... tanbûrlar 'udlar safâ-agar dilnüvâz sazlar çaldurub nev' nev' serdârlarile öyle hoş dil u mesrûr oldılar*).[9] The second volume of the *Hünernâme* (1588), too, has multiple references to hunting banquets that Süleyman I enjoyed. Once, in the hunting garden previously on the location of the Süleymaniye complex near the Old Palace, the sultan shot a huge stag, a *tag sığın* with an arrow. Blood poured from its head, and the animal dropped dead. After a (nervous) suspense, one of the shepherds in attendance stepped in to slaughter the *sığın*, and its meat was "weighed in the scale of benevolence" and "sold with the measure of a bow": *keffe'-i ihsânda terâzû-yı kemânla satıldı.* Then, its (angel-conquered) heart was roasted (*kebab*) and served to those who had been watching.[10] The accompanying double-folio miniature shows the sultan and his retinue, across from a deer with huge antlers, each with six prongs (indicating he was more than five years old), enclosed within red railings. Outside the fence is a herd of roe deer, including their young as well as rabbits, all running free.[11] This account concludes with the verse: "I am the one who hunts lions, I make *kebab* the deers I hunt." The same lines were introduced earlier, at the author's first reference to Süleyman's absorption in the hunt.[12] In another instance, the *Hünernâme* mentions that when the sultan was hunting at Edirne, the game was so abundant that the locals were allowed to have a share of it; they overcame the grief of all the blood that had been shed by turning it into wine and were overjoyed as each one enjoyed *kebab* (*şikârât halka mübâh olup her kimesne mahzûz ve behremend oldılar ve her biri bir küşte üzerine yükleyib hûn-ı cigerden şarâb idüp kebâbdan kâm ü murâd buldular*).[13]

In addition to various references to the Ottoman royal hunt in the period *şehnâme*s, in 1599–1600 the Ottoman bureaucrat-historian Mustafa Âli writes about the pleasures of eating game in his *Tables of Delicacies Concerning the Rules of Social Gatherings*.[14] He notes that "it is well known to the nations, and both the humble and the respectable are agreed, that the food of hunting is a delicious, sweet morsel such as nourishes the soul, and that neither the hungry nor the satiated will ever be filled by those delicious tidbits." He continues to name the game animals, the meat of which was licit to eat (more below).

Then, it is Mustafa Sâfî, *imam* and confidant (as well as chronicler) to Ahmed I (r.1603–17), who reveals much about various aspects of the royal hunt as it was practiced in the early seventeenth century. His *Zübdetü't-Tevârih* abounds in accounts of banqueting. Thus immediately after his enthronement at the age of thirteen, we find Ahmed I frequently hawking in the royal gardens of Istanbul.[15] In palace parlance, such hunting was referred to as *yimeklik*, which literally means "things intended as food" or "to be eaten," because it produced fresh birds for the sultan's table. Mustafa Sâfî mentions *yimeklik* several times,[16] and makes it clear that it sometimes involved staying overnight: *manzûr olan bağçeye yimeklik tarîki üzre ki, ehl-i sarây ıstılâhı üzre zihâb ü iyâbı bir günlük veya bir gün bir gicelik seferden 'ibâretdür.*[17] Once, after a hunting party, the sultan entertained himself in the company of his select courtiers (*nedîmân-ı hâss ve bendegân-ı pür-ihlâs*) with exceptional conversation and revelry (*sohbet-i şâhâne ve 'işret-i sâlihâne*).[18] The next day, after the morning prayers, the party continued with (a large amount of) good food and amity (*hân-ı nimet küşâde ve sofra-ı bî-minmet nihâde olub ta'âm-ı ma'a hazar tenâvülünden kaza-ivatar olunduktan sonra*), and then resumed hunting.[19] It was spring and the sultan was at a royal garden called *Rumili Bahçesi*.

In another instance in Istanbul, when they were in the vicinity of 'Alem Dağı, they rested after some sight-seeing, ate delicious food (*tenâvül-i et'ime-i pâkize-i pür-lezzet*), and continued hunting yet again.[20] Similarly, when they visited a place called Sıra, hidden in the mountains in the vicinity of Üsküdar, they enjoyed a feast of pleasant things to swallow (*ta'âm-ı hôşgüvâr*) and sweet drinks (*şerbet-i tayyibetü'l-âşâr*). On such occasions Mustafa Sâfî admires and praises the cooks and the sweet-makers time and again.[21]

He also talks about the shortage of food and the preparation of food during hunting parties. In September 1605, slightly less than a year and half after Ahmed I's enthronement, the royal party had set out for *yimeklik* at Haramideresi, the first way station westward.[22] They did not stay there, however, and moved on to Çatalca with the intention of moving even further on to Edirne. This unplanned excursion caught the hunting organization unawares and ill-equipped, for they had taken neither enough food (*zer ü zevâd* and *zâhire/zehâir*) nor any proper clothing with them. That night, a carriage was sent back to Istanbul, and at noon the next day three cart-loads of provisions arrived. It was only then that the party moved on to Edirne. As they travelled fast, staying only in four staging stations instead of the usual twelve, the attendants did not have any time to cook or eat. They moved so fast from Çatalca to Silivri, and then to Çorlu that the sultan's attendants found the opportunity to eat only during their fourth stop, at Burgos [Lüleburgaz].[23] This was Ahmed I's first visit to Edirne.

Birds, Hares, Deer, and Boar

The royal hunting parties would take cock and hen pheasant, quail, partridge, wild duck of all species, wild geese and even bustard, so as to provide delicacies for the banquet as well as plumes of cranes and herons for turban aigrettes. In spring 1611, at a time when the gardens and the imperial lodge at Davudpaşa were being renovated, the sultan moved into a tent together with his boon companions. As they hunted, says Mustafa Sâfî, artists in the sultan's retinue captured the game on paper. (It should be noted that, in addition to many hunting scenes compiled in royal illustrated histories, there are also numerous single-page drawings of both hunting birds and game birds in the miniature albums of this period.[24]) Only six birds (six "wings," as Mustafa Sâfî puts it) were taken on that occasion.[25] He adds that according to the registers that were kept, over the autumn and winter of 1611 altogether 110 "wings" were captured in hunting parties at Davudpaşa, Rumeli, Istavroz, Kandil, Göksu, Haramideresi, Beşiktaş, and Kağıthane.[26] He implies that there might have been much more, but that it was not possible to register or to capture all these in painting; he also makes an effort to justify this frustratingly meagre number by repeatedly saying that although the sultan had been out to hunt every day (in other words, although he tried his utmost), it had been a tough winter.

There are also accounts of wild boar chases in those years. The peasants of several villages in the vicinity of Üsküdar were conscripted into service as drovers, and taken to the parks at Beykoz, to the mountain water source called Kayış Pınarı, or to the commons (*ziyâretgâh*) called Ali Bahâdır.[27] When the animals, namely rabbits, foxes, deer, wolves, bears, and wild boar (*har-gûş, rûbâh, ahû-yu sünbül-giyâh, gürg ü hırs ü hûk-ı rûy-siyâh*), were being driven into circles as the drovers kept shouting and yelling (*hâ vü hû ve nâ're-i yâhû*), the sultan arrived with his huntsmen and ordered them to shoot with their muskets. Mustafa Sâfî immediately interjects that the sultan himself used only bow and arrow. In the end, he reports, the party succeeded in hunting a few wild boars "with spears and arrows." There is no mention of any subsequent feasts in this or other accounts of wild boar chases. No on-site pictures were mentioned either.

It is understood that not only an artist but also a scribe was appointed to document the game taken during special parties. Thus, 18 musk-scented deer, 150 baby rabbits, 40 vigilant foxes, and a few ferocious wolves were recorded during a drive at Çömlek.[28] At another time, at Kurdkayası 12 deer, 127 rabbits, 33 foxes, and one "fierce" wolf were hunted.[29] Both these drives were part of a hunting spree in Edirne in the winter of 1612–13. This was the second trip that Ahmed I took to Edirne, just seven years after the first in 1605. The author notes that in the period January12–March 31, a personal attendant of the sultan, Haseki Hüseyin, recorded in his register a total of four large-scale drives and 17 private parties.[30] The first drive was on February 10, 1613 (Zilhicce 18, 1022), at Çömlek;[31] the second was on February 21 (Muharrem 1, 1022), at Kurdkayası.[32] The aforementioned numbers pertain to these two drives. Although the deer, rabbits, foxes, and lone wolf bagged at Kurdkayası added up to 173, Mustafa Sâfî explains that these were only the numbers submitted to the sultan and recorded in a register, *haseki defteri*, so-called after the *bostancı* in charge.[33] The actual number of rabbits turned over to the attendants on the way to the hunting lodge at Çömlek amounted to more than 150. He added that 365 was the total number of the game captured in these two drives. The third drive was at Karaağaç, on March 9 (Muharrem 17, 1022). The total number of deer, rabbits, foxes, and wolves taken came to 144. The fourth and final drive in the winter of 1613 was again at Kurdkayası on March 21 (Muharrem 29, 1022). It yielded 60 game animals. Later, Mustafa Sâfî gives the total bag for all four drives, recorded in the official register, as 915; he also adds that including those taken away by the peasants or submitted in search of favors, this number would have reached 1,200. As noted earlier, Ahmed I also spent days hawking along the Tunca, and those birds (geese, ducks, partridge, and storks) that just the sultan himself captured came to a total of 100 wings.[34] Relying just on this one carefully kept register, Mustafa Sâfî does not really bother to record the numbers of game taken elsewhere–not even when he himself was an eye-witness. Only once, he counts some forty carcasses that court attendants piled up in the courtyard of the Privy Chamber.[35] All in all, these are quite unassuming numbers when compared to the hundreds and thousands that were recorded over the last quarter of the century.

From 1650 to 1681, Ahmed I's grandson Mehmed IV (famous as Avcı: "the Hunter") participated in at least 50 hunting expeditions—mostly in the vicinity of Edirne and beyond. In several cases, huge numbers are listed by his chronicler Abdurrahman Abdi.[36] On one occasion in April 1666, for example, 2,200 rabbits and eighty foxes were killed.[37] During a three-day span in November 1667, the sultan engaged in battue hunting, killing ninety-four deer, four stags, three roebucks, and three wolves, as well as in sedan-chair hunting, where he took eleven deer and three wild boars.[38] In April 1668, two battue expeditions netted seven roebucks, seventeen stags, six wolves, and two lynxes.[39] In February 1670, 364 rabbits were taken in five days,[40] and in April 143 roebucks in two days.[41] These numbers can be compared to those for hunter-kings to the east and west. K'ang-hsi (r. 1661–1722) notes that since his childhood, with bow or gun, he had killed in the wild 135 tigers, 20 bears, 25 leopards, 20 lynxes, 14 tailed *mi* deer, 96 wolves, and 132 wild boars, as well as hundreds of ordinary stags and deer. He then says: "How many animals I killed when we formed the hunting circles and trapped the animals within them I have no way of recalling."[42]

It is worth noting that Abdurrahman Abdi Paşa does not record even a single hunting banquet in detail. Instead, he makes passing reference to various feasts following hunting parties. For example, he mentions the banquet (*ziyâfet*) of the grand vizier at Çardak woods.[43] Then at Tâvûslı, he notes that the sultan did not engage himself in any diversion whatsoever after eating (*ba'de 't-tâ'âm aslâ meks ü ârâm itmeyüp*).[44] Mehmed IV is frequently reported as having his meal in his tent. It seems that these were private and fast lunches or dinners (which, apparently, were also called *yimeklik*). He enjoyed one such discreet meal on the hills known as the Ergene woods (*yimeklik olup*);[45] at another time, near Zağra-ı Atîk, when the roayl party drove the woods at Sülüklü and reached the feasting camp, they ate such convenience food (*korusu sürülüp yimekliğe gelince*).[46] On yet another occasion, when he was at Kapucıköy, we are told that the sultan chose not to eat in his tent, but in the humble dwelling of a poor man (*bir fâkirün hâneciğini teşrif... hâtırcığını taltîf... ta'âmı anda tenâvül*).[47] At Karacabeğ, we are told that the sultan ate some of the roasted partridge (*keklik kebabı*) served for him and then sent the rest to his grand vizier.[48] Only a few times was there a great hunting feast (*azîm şikâr safâsı*).[49]

Hunting and Banqueting in the Winter of 1612–1613

Back in the early seventeenth century, Ahmed I's second unplanned excursion to Edirne seems to have found the sultan in a more enthusiastic mood. In December 1612, the sultan moved to the hunting parks at Davudpaşa for the winter and heart-charming spectacles (*nakl-i zimistânî ve seyr-i dilsitânî*) and busied himself with hunting during the day as well as with pleasures at night (*gündüz şikâr ve gice serîr-i sa'âdetde karâr üzre iken.*)[50] Towards the end of the month, while hunting daily in the vicinity of Davudpaşa (but sleeping in his comfortable bed in the evenings), the sultan once more on the spur of the moment decided to visit Edirne yet again, but this time with the intention to hunt in the grand manner of his ancestors. Not only the hunting establishment and his best men, his privy chamber, and his boon companions, but also the harem including the young princes, the grand vizier, and other Imperial Council members accompanied the sultan.[51] All along the way, the sultan performed various deeds of chivalry (*merdlik*) and religiosity during the day. In the evenings they gathered for entertainments. However, no feasting is mentioned.[52]

Hunting aids, including hunting dogs (*tazî, kilâb*) and cats (*pars nev'i-den Türk tazî*, which could mean cheetahs), as well as a boat (*sefîne-i sebükseyr*), which moved so rapidly on the Tunca river that it was regarded as a marvel of its time (*sürat-i hareketde misâl-i zü'l-cehâneyn bir tayr olan kâyık-ı nâdiru'l-'asr*) were brought up from the capital. The Istanbul-style hunting parties (i.e., with low-flying hawks in the royal gardens) that the sultan enjoyed in Edirne over a period of four months climaxed in four ferocious drives. Two major feasts were thrown during these parties, and they shed great light on Ottoman royal hunting banquets. Mustafa Sâfî recorded them carefully and enthusiastically, though it may be assumed that he omitted the improper, the offensive, or the provocative from his account.

These exclusive celebration feasts for elite guests may well have resulted in a certain relaxation of social mores. Perhaps precisely because of that, Mustafa Sâfî is very keen to emphasize again and again that Ahmed I did not neglect his religious obligations at any time during these hunting parties.[53] We also know that communal—and sometimes very heavy—consumption of alcohol was the norm in such courtly gatherings. Nizâm al-Mulk, chief counselor to the Seljuqs, speaks of Sasanian monarchs' penchant for combining the chase with drinking and womanizing and warns that too much drinking in particular could bring ruin to the state.[54] But despite such concerns, and the even more basic Islamic injunctions against alcohol, many Muslim courts, including the Ghaznavids and others, took to the field well supplied with wine.[55] This was such a frequent occurrence that the royal hunt became identified with good times, even wild times; it came to be viewed as a large, outdoor, floating party.[56] For some this was something to censure, but for others such stories only added to the allure of the royal hunt.[57] As for Ahmed I, given that he had already made a reputation for himself as "the Pious," he is likely to have been consuming only sweetened drinks; and surely, even if this included sweet wines, Mustafa Sâfî was not going to put it on record.

The Banquet at Çömlek/Çölmek

In the winter of 1612–13, the sultan and his retinue explored all the royal hunting gardens (*sebzezâr-ı şikâr*) in the vicinity of Edirne. It often seems that they moved along the Tunca by boat, possibly hawking waterfowl while sight-seeing and enjoying the view.[58] Then they wanted to organize a drive to hunt rabbits, foxes, and deer in the wild, and the sultan ordered the *bostancıbaşı* to find a likely spot with abundant game. The chief gardener was then told to gather the *bostancı*s under his command as well as peasants from villages which had previously participated in drives of this scale and to get there in three days' advance to encircle an area of a few days' distance in perimeter. Together with the hunting attendants, they would then drive the animals to where the sultan would be stationed.[59] The palace and park near Çömlek village, a renowned royal hunting ground (*saydgâh-ı selâtîn-i Âl-i Osman*) since the reign of Murad II, was chosen as the venue. Mustafa Sâfî adds that it had not been in use for some time. In the event, the *bostancıbaşı* did mobilize the peasants to drive all the animals into an oak grove (*mîşezâr*) like a fine sieve.[60]

On the evening of February 12, the sultan and his hunting retinue set out (from Edirne) eight hours after sunset, together with all their hunting birds, dogs, and equipment.[61] Chief of the privy chamber (*odabaşı*) Cafer Ağa, the sword-bearer (*silâhdâr*) and simultaneously barber Muhammed

Ağa, the lackey in charge of costumes (*çuhadâr*) Ahmed Ağa, and the stirrup-holder (*rikâbdâr*) İsmail Ağa were serving as the sultan's close bodyguard. As they marched in the moonlight, they surveyed the area and took steps to block the possible escape routes for the animals.[62] Once more, Mustafa Sâfî notes that Ahmed I did not neglect to perform his morning prayers. The *bostancıbaşı* reported to the sultan about the game that had been fenced in and showed him to his hunting station, where a luxurious tent had been prepared for his comfort. Then, with a *hû vü hâ*, the chase began.[63]

First and foremost they drove the harmful animals, the wolves and foxes. The sultan himself hunted with a bow and arrow (*tîr ü keman*). Later, his companions and hunting staff were allowed to send in the dogs. Finally, the peasants were permitted in; they were to bring whatever was bagged to the sultan and receive their cash gifts in return.[64] Mustafa Sâfî asserts that the main goal of the hunt was to benefit the poor and needy. As noted earlier, the drive at Çömlek yielded 18 deer, 150 rabbits, 40 foxes, and a few wolves.[65]

After the hunt, the sultan moved to the Çömlek hunting lodge (*kasr*) first built by Murad II and then rebuilt and refurbished by Süleyman I. Eulogizing the *kasr* with several couplets, the author goes on to celebrate its pool and fountain. Not only the local water but also the air is praised for its digestive qualities. About the water of the fountain, he goes on to say: "If its taste and flavor were to be described, the candy of Hama (?) has no worth [by comparison] and if it were to be praised in the presence of connoisseurs, the answer would be 'grind its sugar, drink its juice.' It is its light quality which satisfies, not its quantity! Thanks to its perfect digestive [quality] those who eat nearby [at the fountain], will never feel full."[66] Precisely at this point Mustafa Sâfî also notes that all game was brought into the hunting lodge. While writing in his ornate language about the distinctive qualities of the air and water at Çömlek, he seems to have had the impending banquet in mind.

In due order, he mentions that the royal hunter divided up his bag of game among those statesmen who were not present at the the great blood-letting (*bu melhame-i kübrâya nâzır olmayan erbâb-ı devlet*). This was primarily a demonstration of generosity, approval and favor.[67] It was also a virtually obligatory act of royal or lordly redistributionism (as with the apportioning of all movable booty, as well as immovable sources of revenue, including especially the land, in the form of fiefs or prebends). Hence, too, it was ritualized into a dispensation of royal favor, an essential tool of political culture. As much as it was a valuable reward for dependants and a powerful gesture in the cycle of reciprocity, helping to develop and reinforce patronage networks,[68] it also served as a pointer to the importance of consuming game at elite tables. Venison was the most desirable of all.[69] Thus, first the grand vizier and other viziers, followed by the two military judges for Rumeli and Anadolu, all received deer (*âhû*) and rabbits (*hargûş*). Subsequently, the members of the harem and the privy chamber, the attendants of the imperial treasury, the pantry and the stores, as well as the wardrobe (*kilerli* and *seferli*), received their share of the bag.

Finally, it was time to enjoy the food itself (*ba'dehû vakt-i tenâvül-i ta'âm ü gıdadân zemân-i ahz-ı kâm olmagın*).[70] Mustafa Ağa the *silahdâr*— also the sultan's barber—was in command of the feast, and he himself served out the most delicious portions. The menu is not specified. It is rather generically referred to as comprising delicious dishes, sweets, and delicacies (*et'ime-i nefise/ nefâis-i et'ime, hulviyyât-ı nefîse, nefâis-i be-hiyye*). A small portion of each course was tasted according to the prefer-ences of the sultan (*meyl-i tabî'at ve kadr-ı rağbet hasebince her birinden birer mikdâr tenâvül*); however, it is not clear whether it was this style of sampling that he preferred, or the kinds of food that were actually sampled. All leftovers from such delicious plates were then served to his attendants (*ol evânî-i latîfe ve zurûf-ı nazîfe-i huddâm-ı zevi'l-ihtirâm dahî ba'de 'r-ref' tedâvül idüb . . . kendülere i'tâ buyurılan nevâlelerden (211a) istîfâ itdikten sonra*). This was followed by socializing and diversions (*sohbet* and *teferrüç*) until noon prayers the next day. In the sultan's company were his long standing boon companions (*kâim-i ber-pâ olan bî-zebânân ve nüdemâ*).[71]

During this sumptuous feast at Çömlek, the versatile cooks and con-fectioners of the imperial kitchens are said to have served their most artful dishes, which they had prepared the previous night.[72] Given that game is low in fat, a considerable time is necessary for its preparation. Whether deer, birds, or furred animals, it needs to be left hanging for a long time so that the meat becomes tender. Another method of tenderizing is marinating. Grilling or slow cooking also helps to make it more tender. It is possible that such preparations had already been made for the feast in the sultan's tent, i.e., some game may have been previously secured and cured even before the arrival of the royal party. All along, Mustafa Sâfî continues to extol the cooks and sweet-makers. Nevertheless, the food served is repeatedly identified simply as "[main] dishes, sweets, and sweetened drinks" (*yimek, helva, şerbet*). Considerably more information is provided on protocol. We learn, for example, that when a feast was given (*yimek hediye edilirse*), it was ancient law for the chief warder (*kilercibaşı* or *ser-kâr-ı gıda*) and the *ağa*s of his chamber to be in charge. Only if they were unable to take charge, was it up to the sultan's sword-bearer (who was also in charge of the gold dishes) to take over.[73] This was the case at Çömlek.

The sultan returned to Edirne after a day that he spent wandering around and regularly performing the *namaz* near the pool. The next section, an account of a drive at Kurdkayası, also begins with Mustafa Sâfî repeating that the sultan, absorbed in hunting, never neglected to perform the *namaz*.[74] Through such repeated references to Ahmed I's religiosity, Mustafa seems to have been trying to balance the sultan's lust for hunting and partying.

The Banquet at Kurdkayası

For the organization of the subsequent chase at Kurdkayası, the grand vizier Nasuh Paşa stepped in and asked for it to be handed over to him.[75] After all, the chase was an important component of ruling elite relations, military preparations, domestic administration, communications networks, and the search for political legitimacy. The food to be consumed on site was among the three main items on the grand vizier's agenda. In addition to general preparations and provisioning, he was to oversee the preparation of delicious dishes and countless delicacies (*et'ime-i hoş-güvâr* and *nefâis-i lezîze-i bî-şümâr*) for the sultan.[76] The *bostancıbaşı* together with 300 additional *bostancı*s had moved to the hunting ground three or four days earlier. Kurdkayası was one *menzil* away from Edirne. It was a hillock overlooking the plains (*tell-i 'âlî ve bir püşte-i vesî'âtü'l-hâvâli*). There are repeated references to the nearby oak groves.[77] Thousands of peasants from local villages, which since the days of the Ottoman conquest had repeatedly provided manpower for such large-scale battues, drove wild bucks, hares, foxes, jackals, and other wild beasts to the hunting station. Mustafa Sâfî notes that since Süleyman I, animals in the wild (including *sığın*) had not been chased—they had not seen or heard hunters for a very long while.[78] It was icy cold, wet, and snowy in the camping area. Over and over again, Mustafa Sâfî emphasizes the harshness of the environment.

Tents were pitched at the top and the animals were gathered at the foot of the hill, after which the *bostancıbaşı* invited the sultan to the hunting ground.[79] All other viziers and commanders were gathered to watch from another station, out of the sultan's sight. This is a curious arrangement. If it was not due to lack of space at the summit, then it is possible that the sultan was singled out in an attempt at 'heroizing' him. As princely decorum was carefully maintained, the viziers and commanders stayed in their tents and waited for the grand vizier's invitation to the grand banquet.[80] It is worth noting that Mustafa Sâfî grumbles not only about the wind, snow, and frost, but also about the separation of the sultan's tent from the others—what he regards as his separation from the fire place, the "rose garden" of intimate friends. According to Mustafa Sâfî, under the prevailing weather conditions these were unbelievable orders.[81] He adds a couple of words to expound on his own misery. He does not mince his words in complaining about all the hardships, yet in the same breath he also describes the grand vizier's efforts to prepare for the cooking, the talented cooks' and confectioners' energy and enthusiasm, how they mixed work with joy, and the magnificence of what was finally served, all with utmost admiration and delight. He repeatedly says that the grand vizier and other viziers had embarked on these preparations the day before the sultan's arrival.

Three days earlier, it seems, the grand vizier had sent cooking vessels, together with quick and dexterous cooks and sweetmakers, to the site, and had ordered delicious and artful food, sweets, and drinks to be prepared.[82] At this point, the food and drinks destined for the sultan and his company are again listed generically as *nefâis-i et'ime-i lezîze, sanâif-i halâvat,* and *eşribe-i nefîse,* or even more generally as *envâ-ı ta'âm* and *ecnâs-ı nefâis-i lezzet hitâm.* Mustafa Sâfî then mentions the food prepared for the drovers, and in contrast to all previous generalizations, this time he is more specific. In several large cauldrons, the two staple dishes of *pilav* and *zerde* were cooked. Two others, *kalye* and *nehy-i perverde,* which were also prepared in huge amounts, were dishes relatively rare (*nâ-dîde vü nâ-horde*), he says.[83] *Kalye* is a meat stew (ragout) with fruits and vegetables, while the latter, *nehy-i perverde*, requires some explanation (see below).[84]

Eight hours after sunset, the *bostancıbaşı* announced the sultan's arrival in the company of the chief of the black eunuchs Hacı Mustafa, the chief of the privy chamber Cafer Ağa, the sword-bearer Muhammed Ağa, the lackey in charge of sultan's costumes Ahmed Ağa, and the stirrup-holder İsmail Ağa. As soon as they arrived the sultan performed his *namaz*. Mustafa Sâfî celebrates the sultan's perseverance in the face of hardship with several couplets.

The description of the sultan's tent, as well as of the glittering tableware made out of gold and silver and encrusted with precious gems and pearls, is quite exceptional.[85] After resting for a while, the meal was served. The food is once more described in general terms: delicious dishes and sweets (*et'ime-i hoş-güvâr* and *ağdiye-i nefâset-medâr*). The porcelain and celadon serving sets, as many as stars in the sky, were equally dazzling.[86] The sultan, seated on a heavenly throne, sampled the various dishes and sweets set out on the lavish table and enjoyed socializing with his *aga*s, *nedim*s, and *musahib*s to the accompaniment of music. The grand vizier received gifts in return for his services.[87] At the same time food was sent out to the other dignitaries and commanders (*et'ime-i şehiyyesinden sofralar irsâl olunub*).[88] By then it was noon and time for prayers.

Then the grand vizier invited Ahmed I to the hunting ground,[89] but before he made a move, first the *odabaşı* and then the *silahdar* were asked to report on the approaching drovers and the game. Leaving the warmth and comfort of the tent and the delicious food waiting to be eaten, the sultan watched his entourage hunting in the blizzard. All along Mustafa Sâfî provides a running commentary on the weather.[90] The author then reflects on the cruelty and the manliness of the hunt, as well as its gifts and virtues. There follows a unique description of the hunt.[91] The sultan himself did not participate in the chase. Later he distributed gold and silver to those who had presented what they had taken, dead or alive. After that it it was supper time.

Mustafa Sâfî sings the praises of the cooks and the sweet-makers. He waxes eloquent about the food prepared by these talented chefs for supper. Although he still uses generic terms such as *nefâis-i et'ime-i hoş-güvâr* and *sanâif-i ağdiye-i çâşnidâr,* he does provide us with some crucial details. He says that these dishes were "prepared" (*ta'biye*) with musk and amber-gris, "cured" (*terbiye*) with selected other roots (*âkâkir-i muteber*), and "cooked" (slowly) over a weak fire (*âteş-i hâdîye*).[92] This description is almost as good as a recipe.[93]

Served on gold dishes and silver plates, the pleasant smells of these dishes perfumed the mind; the odor of pure musk (*miskiyye*) floated over the party. While the sultan sampled everything set out on the lavish table, the grand vizier watched him from a hidden corner of the royal tent, looking for signs of his satisfaction. What he witnessed was the dignified calmness of the sultan.[94] Could it be that the grand vizier was looking for more than signs of the sultan's approval of his efforts to organize the banquet— including, perhaps, indications of whether the young and pious sultan might get intoxicated and lose his self-control? Mustafa Sâfî then highlights the sweet musky drinks that were offered,[95] together with rose-water, ambergris and other perfumes.[96] Those who ate at this sumptous table stood up and prayed to God and for the sultan in gratitude. They then performed the *namaz.* Four hours after sunset, the sultan returned to the hunting lodge at Çömlek.

Drives at Karaağaç and Kurdkayası, and More Banquets the Following Winter

After he narrates the sultan's return to Edirne, Mustafa Sâfî goes on to give a general account of the sultan's hunting parties during his stay in Edirne. The two other drives, one at Karaağaç and the other again at Kurdkayası, are not described in detail. He only notes the aforementioned dates and the total number of game, which appears to have been copied from the registers kept by Haseki Hüseyin, the former *gulâm-ı bostanî* and *mülâzım-ı rikâb-ı sultânî.* Meanwhile, he continues to relate the reasons for the royal hunt.[97] Strikingly, the views he expresses here are quite similar to the ones that I have found in an early seventeenth-century manuscript from the Topkapı Palace collection. This is an Ottoman Turkish translation of a medieval Arabic text, *'Umdat al-Mulûk,* under the title *Tuhfetü'l-mülûk ve's-selatin* (The Gift of Kings and Sultans).[98] Dedicated to Ahmed I, the illustrated manuscript comprises three sections, namely (1) Hippiatry; (2) Hippology and Horsemanship; and (3) Hunting. It seems to have been compiled and prepared around 1610, at a time when hunting was emerging not only as martial substitute, but also as a personal passion for the young sultan.[99]

Back in the winter of 1612–13, the sultan kept hunting on the way to Istanbul, but no banqueting is recorded.[100] Next summer, he was back in his daily routine in the capital. On August 20, 1613 (Receb 4, 1022), we find him travelling from Çatalca to the hunting lodge at Halkalı, where the royal party was going to spend the night. This trip took an hour or two with the royal ladies and princes in their carriages (*harem-i muhterem arabaları ile*).[101] The next day, after eating there (*mikdâr-ı kabûl tenâvül buyurduktan sonra*) the royal party returned to Çatalca where they were going to celebrate the holy night of *Regaib*.[102] More hunting took place at the Çatalca and Halkalı hunting parks during their ten-day stay.[103] Mustafa Sâfî notes the scarcity of game and relates the sultan's positive interpretation: no hunt meant their emancipation from its sins.[104] The same year, in the holy month of Ramazan (October-November 1613), they moved to Davudpaşa where banquets and other entertainment took place, but no hunting.[105]

Later that year, the sultan went on his third Edirne expedition. The royal party left Istanbul on November 22, 1613.[106] As usual, there was hunting at and around many of the way stations. At Burgaz a drive was organized. At lunch time (*kuşluk*), they were served abundant and delicious food, as well as bread that was soft and white; everything had been prepared by the mobile kitchen.[107] Arriving in Edirne on December 4, the court stayed there until February 1614.[108] This time Mustafa Sâfî was ordered to narrate the sultan's princely activities in verse.[109] He composed a *kasîde* which celebrates Ahmed's arrival in Edirne. Occasionally, it dwells on special moments of pleasure, ranging from boat trips to hunting parks to banquets. It also mentions a feast thrown by the grand vizier.[110] The food, served in celadon dishes, was beyond description to those who did not sample it, says Mustafa Sâfî. The sweetmeats were perfumed either with musk (*mümessek*) or with anbergis (*mu'anber*). Then came sweet fruit stews, compotes which were beyond description, and various pure sherbets. Entertainments followed:

Çü vakt-ı çâşt- oldı sadr-ı a'zam
Çeküb ni'met berây zayf-ı mükerrem

Getürdi mâide sultân önine
Ki 'akl irmez anun aslâ sonına

Nefâis kim anı vasf idemez dil
Anı zevk itmeyene vasf müşkil

Olur vasfında anun 'akl kâsır
K'anı fehm eylemekdir zevka dâir

Çekildi cümle sahn-ı mertebânı
Ki tefrîh eyler ol rûh-ı revânı

Gelüb etbâk-ı hulviyyât yekser
Mümessek kimi, kimisi mu'anber

Dökildi âhirinde cins-i hoş-âb
Ki kemm ü keyfî vasfı oldı nâyâb

İçildi gûne gûne şerbet-i nâb
Olundı teşne diller cümle sîrâb

Tamâm oldı çü fasl-ı pân-ı ni'met
Açıldı bâb-ı hamd ü şükr ü minnet

Pes andan sonra şüst ü şûy oldı
Nedîmân içre güft ü gûy oldı

İdüb her biri bir dürlü zarâfet
Virür ol meclis-i inse tarâvet

Nehy-i Perverde, the Forbidden Food

With regard to the food that was served to the hunting attendants and commoners (including both peasant and poor) who had participated in the chase
as I have already noted, Mustafa Sâfî says that it consisted of *pilav, zerde*
and *kalye*—"a dish they see very seldom" he adds—as well as something
called *nehy-i perverde*.[111] Now *nehy* (A.) means "prohibited," and *perverde*
(P.), which literally means nourished or cured, appears to have been a kind
of sweet fruity dessert.[112] Since it was "prohibited," it is very likely that it
was sweetened not with sugar or honey but with grape juice (*şıra*, which
would acquire an alcoholic content through fermentation, eventually ending
up as *şarap* [wine]).

What, then, was this thing that they ate, and which Mustafa Sâfî sees
fit to refer to (in quasi-biblical terms) as "forbidden food?" Did wine really
have something to do with it? Why should it have been *nehy* if indeed it
was only unfermented grape juice that went into it? And was it only the
hunting attendants and drovers to whom it was served, or could the sultan's
imam and confidant have been passing over its presence at the royal table?
Unfortunately, that is all that Mustafa Sâfî has to say about the rare and the
extraordinary, that is to say both the *kalye* and the *nehy-i perverde*.[113]

A clue for the *perverde* comes from a fifteenth-century medical treatise,
Tabîb İbn-i Şerîf's *Yâdigâr*. *Perverde-i hısrım*, a cure for the eyes, is explained in the text as an amalgam of spices diluted in sour, unripe grape
juice (*koruk*).[114] It is understood that garlic may also have been an ingredient of such a mixture (*perverde-i sevm*). A menu of the 1539 circumcision
festival provides us with another clue. Among the twenty tables of desserts
and sweets that were served after dinner on the night of the henna ritual,
*perverde*s of carrot [jam], squash, and quince were listed together with mar-
malades, jams, puddings, preserves, and condiments.[115] Meanwhile, *kalye*
made with quince (*ayva kalyesi*) was listed among the main servings.[116]

Some of the dishes listed in the 1539 banquet book are to be found in
the cookbook of Muhammed bin Mahmûd Şirvanî, written in the first half
of the fifteenth century.[117] Based on Al-Bağdadî's *Kitabü 't-tabih mine
'l-et 'ime fî kable 't-tıbb* of 1226–27, it includes two dishes, *tuffahiye* and
seferceliye, the recipes for which mention *perverde* as a term denoting fruits
cooked with sugar.[118] (Both of these medieval cookbooks were once part

of the Topkapı Palace collections.) The dishes in question differ only by their main ingredient: the first is a dish prepared with apples and the second with quinces. For every two *okka*s of apples or quinces (pure and sweet), 300 *dirhem*s of sugar, 150 *dirhem*s of almonds, 100 *dirhem*s of dates, and an *okka* of mutton, lamb, or poultry were added. First the meat would be cooked to become *kalye*, then 250 *dirhem*s of sugar would be melted in a pot, and 200 *dirhem* of fruits would be cooked in this sugar (*ol şeker içinde perverde bişüre*) to reach a certain consistency. Rose water would be gradually added to dilute the mixture and then cooked again to reach *perverde* thickness. This would be repeated three times. Then the fruits would be taken out of the dish one by one. The meat, taken out of its juice and added to the sugary mixture, would be caramelized and then left to rest. The remaining *okka* of apples or quinces would be pounded in a wooden mortar, squeezed, and then drained through a cloth (*astar*). The pot used to cook the meat would be cleaned, and the apple or pear juice poured in. All the almonds would be finely chopped, one hundred *dirhem*s of them placed in the pot, and the meat and sugar paste (still called *perverde*) added. Then the remaining fruits would be cut into pieces and added, as well as some saffron, diluted in rose water, plus fifteen *dirhem*s of starch, also diluted in rose water. Dates, halved and seeded, and half a seed of musk, diluted in rose water, would also be added, and the whole dish would be salted. Fifty *dirhem*s of sugar would be pounded, added to chopped up almonds, some more misk would be diluted in rose water. The meat would be topped with apples or pears and sprinkled with rose water and sugared almonds.

Mustafa Sâfî's repeated references not to *kebab* (skewered meat) or *külbastı* (grilled meat) but to *kalye*, a meat stew with vegetables and fruits, suggest that they were eating "marinated" meat. Furthermore, the stew in question was not *yahni* (also a meat dish but cooked only with onion or garlic and sometimes with chickpeas), but *kalye*.[119] This further reinforces the idea that there was an emphasis on curing meat in fruit juices. An eighteenth-century cookbook by a Mevlevî dervish gives recipes for marinating.[120] Certainly wine or any other liquid containing alcohol is an impermissible medium for marinating meat. Neither could it be used to cook with or in. However, unripe grapes or their juice or reduced juice would all be used as souring agents. In contrast, grape molasses, produced by boiling down grape juice, served as a sweetener.

The pious Muslim believer was enjoined to avoid alcohol completely, but those who wanted to consume it could resort to a variety of excuses. Thus for some, wine that was diluted or boiled was acceptable. Hence there could be yet another explanation for *nehy-i perverde*. There is the possibility that *nehy-i perverde* referred to some red wine punch marinated with fruits and flavored with spices which they drank warm at the Ottoman court.[121] It would certainly be welcomed in the bitter cold that prevailed during some of these hunting parties. Elsewhere, Mustafa Sâfî refers to various royal sherbets, made from fruit juices, extracts of flowers, or herbs mostly combined with sugar and water to form a syrup that was later thinned with water, ice, or even snow. He notes that when consumed, such sherbets prepared those of manly posture for freedom (towards pure love). Could this be a euphemism for intoxication? Food and drinks being consumed, happiness prevailed, he says, and they moved on:

> *İçildi gûne gûne şerbet-i hâss*
> *Ki ihzâr eylemiş ol merdi ihlâs*

> *Yenildi et'ime şerbet içildi*
> *Sa'âdetle turub andan göçüldü*[122]

There is more than a sense of innuendo to these verses about playful relaxation. In some sherbet recipes the ingredients are diluted in wine vinegar, suggesting intoxicating qualities.[123] The whole complex field of Islam and wine consumption cannot really be tackled within the limits of this study.[124] I can only conclude this section by pointing to a reference to "uncooked" and therefore also "cooked" wine in a story in Firdausi's *Shahname* (Book of Kings), the monumental epic written around AD 1000, and repeatedly copied and adapted also by the Ottomans. It recounts the conflict between Esfandyar, a king's son, and the champion and hero, Rostam.[125] Prior to battle they converse, and Esfandyar says:

> "There is no point in our boasting any more
> About our countless victories in war;
> Enough of who won what, and who was killed;
> The day's half done, we need our stomachs filled!

Let them bring food for us, and while we eat
No one's to talk of victory or defeat!"
As Rostam ate the lamb they brought him there
His appetite made all others stare;
Esfandyar said, "Serve him with uncooked wine,
Let it affect him while we sit and dine,
And when the wine has made his tongue grow loose
We'll hear him chatter about King Kavus!"
The steward brought a cup in which a boat—
Or so it seemed—could have been set afloat.

This takes me to another problem area, the relationship between game and canonically lawful eating. The Hanafi *madhhab* followed by the Ottomans recognized a relatively straightforward list of *halal* and *haram* animals for purposes of consumption.[126] We also know that the royal hunters were keen to set free all *haram* game that was captured alive (*me'kûlü'l-lâhm olmayan şikârları âzâd itmeğile*).[127] The observations of Julien Bordier, squire to the French ambassador to Istanbul (B*aron* de *Salignac*, 1604–12), regarding the fate of wolves and jackals (and more generally of all hunted game) are interesting because the author touches upon an issue that is known to have confronted Muslim hunters since the time of the Prophet. "Some wild animals are distributed among the non-Muslim slaves," Bordier says, "for the Turks only rarely eat venison, and then mainly of such animals that have been [have had their throat] cut by human hands, so as to allow their blood to flow, following in this the rules of Judaism."[128] So according to this interpretation of Koranic law, the hunter was (is) subject to rules regarding the ritual slaughter of captured game in order to preserve the lawfulness, the *halal* nature, of his consumption.

Furthermore, while Europeans hunted with muskets, as already indicated the Ottoman elite did not go shooting with firearms. In fact, Bordier notes not only that the game in Turkey was very abundant, but also that it was almost domesticated because Muslims did not hunt by shooting.[129] According to Mustafa Sâfî, and also as witnessed by Bordier, Ahmed I (like his predecessors) was dedicated to the low-flying bird-hunt even during a chase for larger game. To preserve the lawfulness of consuming the hunted animal, they had to refrain from killing the game on the spot and then picking it up dead. Instead, its throat had to be cut ritually. Clearly, it was much more difficult to refrain from killing any animal outright in the case of hunting by shooting (with muskets), than if the game was hunted with dogs or raptors. Consider the following *fatwas* by Ebussud:[130] Is game shot with a musket or trapped lawful [to eat]? Yes. If the hounds (released with a *besmele*) should happen to kill the game and to eat a bit of it, is the rest lawful [to eat]? No. If the hound should somehow be distracted on its way to the catch, if it should first hide and crouch down in ambush, and then catches up with and kills the animal, is it lawfully edible? No, not if crouching and prowling is not in its nature. If it is a leopard that has been released to a *besmele*, and then the leopard crouches and prowls in ambush prior to killing the prey, is the game lawfully edible? Yes, because crouching is part of the leopard's nature. —These *fatwa*s fully reflect the difficulties and complications of Islamic belief and law in the face of the material realities of hunting. Such difficulties may be said only to have grown with the increasing spread and ascendancy of firearms. Thus Muslim debates about the legitimacy of hunting by shooting did not immediately disappear with the passage of time. In Tunis in the nineteenth century, for example, Sheikh Muhammad Bayram wrote a whole treatise devoted to this issue.[131]

We also need to consider the season in which hunting took place. From the *fatwa* point of view, questions such as "Can we hunt birds and animals at any time?" have tended to be assimilated to the (further) question of "Without any need for food, just for pleasure and enjoyment?"[132] What was especially at issue was the reproduction cycle in the wild. In Europe, June was traditionally the "fence month" for red deer, when hinds dropped their calves and the herds of deer were left undisturbed by hunting or any other interference. This period was the medieval equivalent of a closed season.[133] Aristocratic hunting differed from commoners' hunting in observing the "fence month," the season of non-hunting or not disturbing the red deer. It could be argued that the imposition of a closed season is not a technique of hunting, but that it is certainly part of an aristocratic approach, ethos, or methodology in a wider sense. The other side of the coin is just as much a class-based notion of the best seasons for hunting specific animals.[134]

Visualizing the Banquet

Despite some fascinating puzzles that remain, Mustafa Sâfî's descriptions of the feasts, and especially of the second one described above, remove all previous uncertainties regarding the consumption of game (other than birds) at the Ottoman royal table. As for the manner of cooking and presentation, might we be permitted to assume that it differed little from European practice? There, game birds, such as wild goose, wild duck, wood pigeon, pheasant, partridge, and black and red grouse, were generally cooked whole. It is furred game (including all types of deer, chamois, wild boar, rabbit, and hare) that is likely to have been both prepared for roasting and also (with the flesh removed and chopped up) used in stews (ragouts). The most popular roasting joints were the saddle (or the back), the leg (the haunch), and the shin (or shank). For stews, cuts from the neck, the breast, the head, and the belly, as well as the heart and liver, were preferred. Chopped small(er), lower grade raw meat, as well as any leftovers of already cooked meat, were used together with the bones to make soups. Cutlets were taken from the haunch, shank, sirloin, or the boned saddle. Larger game animals provided juicy spare ribs or chops. The sirloin and the saddle provided good medallion pieces. Offal—the heart, lungs, liver, kidneys, and tongue—could all be made into stews and pies.[135]

I would argue that these vivid textual descriptions were increasingly reflected in a growing dimension of realism in Ottoman miniatures. Thus, whole cooked fowl and stews, grills, and roasts (with great variations in rice dishes) come to be depicted frequently in Ottoman miniatures showing outdoor banquet scenes. Appearing more often from the turn of the seventeenth century, such miniatures start employing an innovative iconography.[136] For example, a remarkable miniature reflecting the social setting of the royal hunt is dated to the last decades of the sixteenth century and bound in a *muraqqa* made in Istanbul for Ahmed I's grandfather[137] (Figure 1). It is a tripartite painting, composed of three horizontal bands, featuring a hunt at the top, a princely garden party in the middle, and a feasting and frolicking group at the bottom.[138] The middle panel depicts an outdoor entertainment with an enthroned young prince and royal lady—perhaps his mother (she appears larger than the prince)—who are being offered food and drink in the company of musicians and dancers. This princely gathering

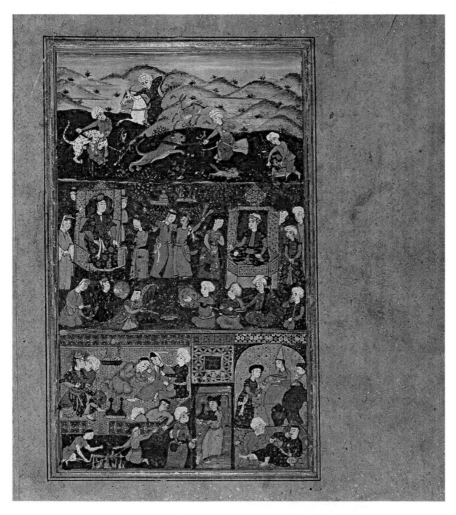

Figure 1. Muraqqa of Murad III : Vienna, Österreische National
Bibliothek, Codex Mixtus 313, 28b. Hunt, a princely party, and feasting.

conforms to the prevalent iconography of banquet scenes in Persian *shah-namas*. What is below it, however, is an imaginative genre scene. In a tavern- or brothel-like setting, servants are filling pitchers of wine from large vats and serving amorous couples. On one side, meat is being roasted on a spit.[139] Other seventeenth-century miniatures featuring outdoor

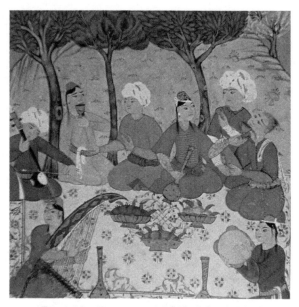

Figure 2a.Tercüme-i Miftâh Cifrü'l-Câmî :
İstanbul, Topkapı Palace Library B. 373 (1597-98), 243b.
Men and women feasting in a garden under trees.

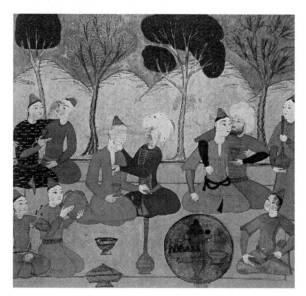

Figure 2b. Tercüme-i Miftâh Cifrü'l-Câmî :
İstanbul, İstanbul University Library, T. 6624.
Men and women feasting in a garden under trees.

banquet scenes, very similar in composition to the middle panel, were mostly compiled in albums (such as the one known as the *Ahmed I Album*), and were possibly made to match with hunting scenes.[140]

This is not a unique occurrence; too many other examples exist for it to be attributed to non-realistic symbolism. Two copies (perhaps a decade apart) of a contemporary manuscript on the occult, *Tercüme-i Miftâh Cifrü'l-Câmî*, also contain miniatures which depict leisurely royal parties where the sultan, the sultana, and her ladies-in-waiting figure prominently. These banquet or outdoor entertainment scenes, based on Persian (and Sasanian) prototypes, may be interpreted so as to support only that part of Shepherd's argument (referred to at the beginning of this article), that has to do with the origins of such scenes in a religious, rather than a secular, iconography. Thus one of the scenes in *Tercüme-i Miftâh Cifrü'l-Câmî* relates to the Apocalyptic punishment, the sending of the wind that, it is believed, would kill all true believers so that in the end only the sinful would suffer the Apocalypse. It is represented by a group of people in frivolous entertainment outdoors, that is to say "in nature"[141] (Figure 2). In the earlier copy, while two women playing a *def* and a *çeng* accompany a third who is dancing, yet another woman serves a drink to a youth seated cross-legged on a throne. In the later copy, the female figures are replaced by males, and the cup-bearer is replaced by a young man reading a book. The second copy was prepared in the reign of Ahmed I. This change may have been introduced to please the pious sultan, or perhaps some in his immediate retinue, on the assumption that he might not have tolerated representations of women, especially in such a setting.

In the *Tuhfetü'l-mülûk ve's-selatin*'s section on hunting, there are several more princely scenes depicting a ruler enthroned and carrying his royal insignia (notably the Persian-style crown), occasionally with a falcon on his wrist. These representations of the royal hunter in the company of his attendants were apparently made to match with representations of ladies partying[142] (Figure 3). These miniatures where the sultan, the sultana, and her ladies-in-waiting figure prominently remind one of those found in the *Tercüme-i Miftâh Cifrü'l-Câmî*.[143] In one group are shown only the sultana and her attendants shooing away flies, while the entertainers are depicted in a separate group. It is possible that the depictions of the sultana (participating in hunting parties) were originally meant to be put together, face to

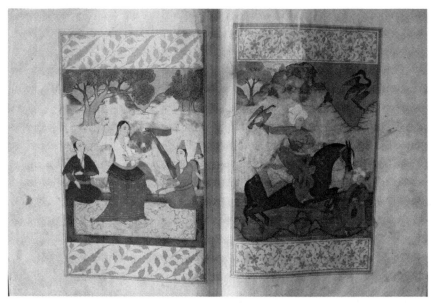

Figure 3a. Tuhfetü'l-mülûk ve's-selâtîn : İstanbul, Topkapı Palace Library
H. 415 (ca. 1610), 240b-241a. Women's outdoor entertainment and hunters.

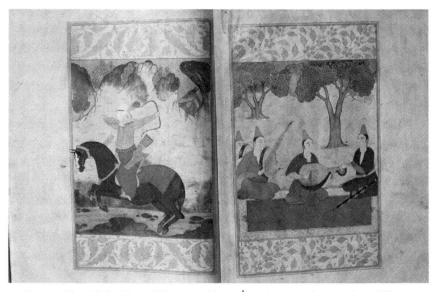

Figure 3b. Tuhfetü'l-mülûk ve's-selâtîn : İstanbul, Topkapı Palace Library
H. 415 (ca. 1610), 241b-242a. Women's outdoor entertainment and hunters.

face, with compositions comprising musicians and dancers, so as to create a more impressive double-folio of playfulness. Unfortunately, all these are in disarray, and there is no way of telling how they were intended to be coupled.[144]

Shepherd identifies three motifs as evidence that such representations do not reflect an earthly feast. These are a diadem, a (wine) cup and a flower (or bowl of fruits, particularly pomegranates). All three are missing from all these various Ottoman miniatures. The Ottoman adoption and translation of established canons of Islamic visual culture into a new representational language cannot be denied or mistaken for anything else.[145] More fundamentally, there is no reason why real-life scenes should not have been fitted into a religious, legitimating framework. Hence, the hunting and banqueting of Ahmed I materializes as a product of culture with an organic relation to the society in which it was produced.

In the *Zübdetü't-Tevârîh,* Mustafa Sâfî seems to have been preparing himself to write a history of Ahmed I's reign, perhaps in the form of an illustrated book of kings. The format of the *Zübdetü't-Tevârîh* is fairly standard and takes after the earlier *şehnâme*s. It is a format developed by Arifi, who was appointed to the post of *şehnâmeci* by Süleyman I around 1550, and enhanced by Seyyid Lokman (in office: 1569–96) as well as by Talikizâde Suphi Mehmed Efendi (1596–99).[146] In the manner of earlier *şehnâmeci*s, Mustafa Sâfî incorporates a wealth of anectodes narrated by those who accompanied the sultan on various hunting occasions. Also in the manner of previous writers of Ottoman official histories, Mustafa Sâfî cites his informants' positions and praises their deeds, thereby underlining the reliability of his own account. The persona of Ahmed I is constructed so as to bring out his prowess, righteousness, or piousness, that is to say, his regal attributes. It is worth noting at this point that Mustafa Sâfî seems to have been quite keen to give a balanced account of the sultan's qualities—hence he represents him as one who never failed to perform *namaz* even during the most strenuous and/or the wildest hunting parties.

Where the author becomes really innovative, however, diverging from previous models and patterns, is when he chooses to narrate Ahmed I's hunting banquets in some detail as part of his efforts to exalt his sovereign. He chooses to reflect on Ahmed I's passion for the hunt not by mimicking the constructs of Firdousi's *Shahname,* but by relating what he himself witnessed.

Perhaps this is also why, when it comes to the banquets, it is not the sultan's customary generosity, but the skills of the cooks and sweetmakers or the organizational talents of the grand vizier that Mustafa Sâfî praises. In this way, these banquets are immediately situated outside pure convention and lifted (or lowered?) to a more realistic plane. Furthermore, the amount of detail that he incorporates on both hunting and feasting practices, including the preparations, the setting, the weather, and the staff employed, is all capable of being easily translated into visual imagery. I would argue that this was actually what he intended. The text as we have it is like a first draft of a *şehname*, needing, apart from more secondary reorganization, only the miniatures of the verbally described scenes to make it explicitly into a genuine book of kings. It is possible that if he had had the time, eventually such images, too, might have been prepared and included.

Notes

1. Richard Almond, *Medieval Hunting* (Phoenix Mill: Sutton Publishing Limited, 2003), p. 16. Almond refers to King Alfonso of Castile (r. 1312–1350) who was echoing the ideas of Xenophon about the similarities between war and hunting. See: Luke Syson and Dillian Gordon, *Pisanello: Painter to the Renaissance Court* (London: National Gallery Co Ltd, 2002), p. 85.

2. *The Ottoman Gentleman of the Sixteenth Century : Mustafa Âli's Mevâ'idü'n-Nefâ'is fî Kavâ'idi'l-Mecâlis "Tables of Delicacies Concerning the Rules of Social Gatherings,"* annotated English translation by Douglas S. Brookes, Sources of Oriental Languages and Literatures 59 (Cambridge, MA: Department of Near Eastern Languages and Civilizations, 2003), p. 38. See also: Muhammed b. Ali b. Süleyman er-Ravendî, *Râhat-üs-Sudûr ve Âyet-üs-Sürûr* II, tr. Ahmet Ateş (Ankara: Türk Tarih Kurumu, 1960), p. 398.

3. There is an impressive literature which deals with topics ranging from the history of leisure and sports to honor, poaching, woodlands, forest laws, popular politics, and hunting. See for example: Roger B. Manning, *Hunters and Poachers: A Social and Cultural History of Unlawful Hunting in England, 1485–1640* (Oxford: Oxford University Press, 1993), esp. chs. 1 and 5; Dan Beaver, "The Great Deer Massacre: Animals, Honor, and Communication in Early Modern England," *Journal of British Studies* 38 (1999): pp. 187–216. The latter, a study of the massacre of several hundred deer in a Gloucestershire chase belonging to the Earl of Middlesex in October 1642, illustrates the social and cultural significance of hunting and of venison in order to emphasise that

the slaughter was a calculated insult to the earl and an attack on his status. This was revenge for the earl's aggressive pursuit of poachers and woodcutters.

4. Thomas T. Allsen, *The Royal Hunt in Eurasian History* (Philadephia: University of Pennsylvania Press, 2006), pp. 196–97.

5. Allsen, *Royal Hunt*, pp. 196–97.

6. For a bibliography on Ottoman hunting: Tülay Artan, "A Book of Kings Produced and Presented as a Treatise on Hunting," *Muqarnas* 25 (2008): pp. 299–330.

7. Dorothy G. Shepherd, "Banquet and Hunt in Medieval Islamic Iconography," in *Gatherings in Honor of Dorothy E. Miner*, ed. Ursula E. McCracken, Lilian M.C. Randall, and Richard H.Randall, Jr. (Baltimore: The Walters Art Gallery, 1974), pp. 79–94 (see p. 80 in particular).

8. At other times, this canon either persists in identifying the gender of the beloved as always female or altogether ignores those texts with an explicitly sexual content. For a recent example of this approach see: Ahmet Atilla Şentürk, "Osmanlı Şiirinde Aşka Dair," *Doğu Batı* 7/26 (2004): pp. 55–68. For a critical evaluation of the prevalent conventional approaches: Kemal Sılay, *Nedim and the Poetics of the Ottoman Court: Medieval Inheritance and the Need for Change*, Indiana University Turkish Studies Series: XIII (Bloomington: Indiana University, 1994); Selim S. Kuru, "Naming the Beloved in Ottoman Turkish Gazel. The Case of İshak Çelebi (d. 1537/8)," in *Ghazal as World Literature*, vol. 2, *From a Literary Genre to a Great Tradition: The Ottoman Gazel in Context*, ed. Angelika Neuwirth, Michael Hess, Judith Pfeiffer, and Boerte Sagaster (Beirut: Ergon Verlag, 2005–2006), pp. 163–73; Selim S. Kuru, "Sex in the Text: Deli Birader's Dâfi'ü'l-gumûm ve Râfi'ü 'l-humûm and the Ottoman Literary Canon," *Middle Eastern Literatures* 10/2 (2007): pp. 157–74. Also see a recent study which compares the gendering tactics in Ottoman texts with those in European examples: Walter G. Andrews and Mehmet Kalpaklı, *The Age of Beloveds: Love and the Beloved in Early-Modern Ottoman and European Culture and Society* (Durham, NC: Duke University Press, 2005).

9. Celalzâde Mustafa, *Tabaqât ül-memâlik ve derecât ül-mesâlik*, in *Geschichte Sultan Süleyman Kanunis von 1520 bis 1557*, ed. Petra Kappert (Wiesbaden: Franz Steiner Verlag, 1981), fol. 205a. For the *Tabaqât* and other primary sources relating to Süleyman I's hunting parties: Melis Taner, "'Power to Kill': A Discourse of the Royal Hunt during the Reigns of Süleyman the Magnificent and Ahmed I" (MA thesis, Sabanci University, 2009).

10. The two volumes of the *Hünernâme* (Book of Talents) contain many references to and several miniatures depicting the hunter-sultan: Topkapı Palace

Museum Library, H. 1523 and H. 1524 respectively. Zekeriya Eroğlu, "Şehnâmeci Lokmân'ın Hüner-nâme'si" (2. cilt,1–154. varak) (MA thesis, İstanbul University, 1998), fol. 88b: *ve melek ü mülükden âvâze'-i âferin gûş-ı câne irişüp ve sîne'-i virânı kebâb kılınup erbâb-ı nezzâreye takdim ve tenâvül buyurdular.* Eroğlu suggests *sağan* for the deer in question, but this is not correct; see: Mesut Şen, "Geyik," in *Av ve Avcılık Kitabı*, ed. Emine Gürsoy-Naskali and Hilal Oytun Altun (İstanbul: Kitabevi Yayınları, 2008), pp. 75–88. In his transliteration of Abdurrahman Abdi Paşa's *Vekâyî'-Nâme*, Fahri Derin, too, has preferred *sağan*: Fahri Ç. Derin, *Abdurrahman Abdi Paşa Vekâyî'-Nâmesi (Osmanlı Tarihi [1648–1682])* (İstanbul: Çamlıca Yayınları, 2008), p. 217 (fol. 70b), p. 273 (fol. 86a), p. 282 (fol. 88b), p. 288 (fol. 90b), p. 321 (fol. 99a), p. 345 (fol. 106a). Only thereafter does he express his doubts, preferring *sığın* and putting *sağan* in parentheses: pp. 346–47 (fol. 106b), p. 353 (fol. 108b).

11. For the miniature: fols. 87b–88a; see: Nurhan Atasoy, *Hasbahçe: Osmanlı Kültüründe Bahçe ve Çiçek* (İstanbul: Koç Kültür Sanat Tanıtım, 2002), p. 231.

12. Topkapı Palace Museum Library, H. 1524, fol. 70a.

13. Topkapı Palace Museum Library, H. 1524, fol. 81a. The accompanying miniature shows the hunt, not the banquet: fol. 80b.

14. *The Ottoman Gentleman of the Sixteenth Century*, pp. 39–40.

15. November 4, 1604, hawking at Rumili Bahçesi: *Zübdetü't-Tevârîh* II, fols. 28a–29a.

16. *Mustafa Sâfî'nin Zübdetü't-Tevârîh'i*, ed. İ. H. Çuhadar (Ankara: Türk Tarih Kurumu Yayınları, 2003), vol. 1, fol. 144b. Mustafa Sâfî mentions a short hunt coupled with picnicking (involving *yimeklik*): *Ol şehen-şâh-ı cihân, ol pâdişâh-ı barr ü berr/ Hazret-i Sultan Ahmed Hân-ı pür-fazl ü hüner/hazretleri bir gün kasd-ı şikâr ve 'azm-i geşt ü güzâr ile bir rahş-ı safâ-bahşe-süvâr ve bir kûhe-i bedî'ü'n-nakş üzre üstüvâr olub sarây-ı 'âmir ıstılâhınca yimeklik diyü tâ'bîr olınan hareket vechi üzre beytûte[t] niyyeti ile 'azîmet idüb.*

17. *Zübdetü't-Tevârîh*, vol. 1, fol. 164a.

18. *Zübdetü't-Tevârîh*, vol. 1, fol. 145b.

19. *Zübdetü't-Tevârîh*, vol. 1, fol. 145b.

20. *Zübdetü't-Tevârîh*, vol. 1, fol. 155a.

21. *Zübdetü't-Tevârîh*, vol. 1, fol. 155b: *anda tabbâhân-ı pâkize-dest ü rû ve âş-pezân-ı tâhir-i bâ vuzû ihzâr itdikleri ta'âm-ı hôş-güvârı tenâvül ve kâsehâ-yı şerbet-i tayyibetü'l-âşârı tedâvül buyurub.*

22. *Zübdetü't-Tevârîh*, vol. 1, fol. 164b. The 1605 Edirne expedition is briefly mentioned also in: *Zübdetü't-Tevârîh*, vol. 2, fols. 183b–184a. See also:

Topçular Kâtibi 'Abdülkâdir (Kadri) Efendi Tarihi, ed. Ziya Yılmazer (Ankara: Türk Tarih Kurumu Yayınları, 2003), p. 610.

23. Documents pertaining to the hunting parties of Mehmed IV that I have studied reveal that the high-ranking hunting attendants received a regular bread allocation. These reflected their rank and status. Likewise, each one received a variety of other foodstuffs. For two such documents, see Başbakanlık Osmanlı Arşivi (BAO) DBŞM 351 (1089) and DBŞM 210 (1070). The latter lists not only bread and meat, but also rice, chickpeas, (broken) wheat, and onions; clarified butter and sesame oil; salt and black pepper, yoghurt, honey, vinegar, and almonds; beeswax.

24. Topkapı Palace Museum Library, B. 408, fol. 24a. A sparrow-hawk (*atmaca*) standing on a perch, H. 2153, fol. 98a; a golden eagle on a perch, H. 2153, fol. 109a; a white falcon (*akdoğan*) on a cushion perch, H. 2154, fol. 17b. See also British Library, Or 2709: p. 21, a goshawk standing on a perch; p. 22, a partridge on a rock. There were also those compiled in albums: Topkapı Palace Museum Library, H. 1263, fol. 17a, H. 2164, fols. 7a, 9b, 10b, 13b, 22b, 44a, 52b.

25. *Zübdetü't-Tevârîh*, vol. 1, fol. 151b: *bâz-ı 'âli pervazlar ile aldıkları altı cenâh şikârın keyfiyyet-i saydın ve anların sûret-i zabt u kaydın ahsen-i tâ'bîr ile beyân ve ebyen-i tefsîr ile takrîr u 'ayân idüb.*

26. *Zübdetü't-Tevârîh*, vol. 1, fol. 148b.

27. *Zübdetü't-Tevârîh*, vol. 1, fol. 156a ff.

28. *Zübdetü't-Tevârîh*, vol. 2, fol. 208b: *onsekiz re's âhû-yı müşk-bû ve yüz elli hargûş-ı rübûde-hûş ve kırk rûbâh-ı bâ-intibâh ve birkaç gürg-i sütürg bulunub.* This last adjective has elsewhere been mistakenly transcribed as *sütrük* or *setürg.*

29. *Zübdetü't-Tevârîh*, vol. 2, fol. 223a: *on iki re's âhû ve otuz üç rûbâh ve yüz yigirmi yedi hargûş ve bir gürg-i sütürg alınmışdur.*

30. *Zübdetü't-Tevârîh*, vol. 2, fols. 225b–226a.

31. *Zübdetü't-Tevârîh*, vol. 2, fols. 204a–211b.

32. *Zübdetü't-Tevârîh*, vol. 2, fols. 211b–229a.

33. *Zübdetü't-Tevârîh*, vol. 2 , fol. 223a.

34. *Zübdetü't-Tevârîh*, vol. 2, fol. 227a.

35. *Zübdetü't-Tevârîh*, vol. 2, 203a. For the numbers of animals captured during the third hunting trip to Edirne: *Zübdetü't-Tevârîh*, vol. 2, 359a.

36. Fahri Ç. Derin, *Abdurrahman Abdi Paşa Vekâyî'-Nâmesi*, pp. 224, 273, 288, 336, 337.

37. *Abdurrahman Abdi Paşa Vekâyî'-Nâmesi*, fol. 72b.

38. *Abdurrahman Abdi Paşa Vekâyî'-Nâmesi*, fol. 86a.

39. *Abdurrahman Abdi Paşa Vekâyî'-Nâmesi*, fol. 90b.

40. *Abdurrahman Abdi Paşa Vekâyî'-Nâmesi*, fol. 103b.

41. *Abdurrahman Abdi Paşa Vekâyî'-Nâmesi*, fol. 104a.

42. Jonathan D. Spence, *Emperor of China: Self-Portrait of K'ang-hsi* (New York: Vintage Books, 1974), p. 9.

43. *Abdurrahman Abdi Paşa Vekâyî'-Nâmesi*, fol. 38a.

44. *Abdurrahman Abdi Paşa Vekâyî'-Nâmesi*, fol. 54b.

45. *Abdurrahman Abdi Paşa Vekâyî'-Nâmesi*, fol. 62a.

46. *Abdurrahman Abdi Paşa Vekâyî'-Nâmesi*, fol. 85b.

47. *Abdurrahman Abdi Paşa Vekâyî'-Nâmesi*, fol. 61a.

48. *Abdurrahman Abdi Paşa Vekâyî'-Nâmesi*, fol. 66a.

49. *Abdurrahman Abdi Paşa Vekâyî'-Nâmesi*, fol. 87a.

50. *Zübdetü 't-Tevârîh*, vol. 2, fols. 184b–185a.

51. The *Dârü's-sa'âde* unit under their chief el-Hâc Mustafa Ağa moved two days before the rest of the sultan's retinue. On 31 December (Zilkade 8, 1021), the sultan started on his way. Included in his entourage were palace attendants such as the taster (*çâşnigîr*) as well as some of his royal guards, the *sipâhiyân* and the *silâhdârân*. Among those dignitaries, both in office and retired, who accompanied him were the *şeyhülislam* Mevlânâ Muhammed Efendi, the instructor (*muallim*) of the princes Mevlânâ Ömer, the chief royal physician Mevlânâ Musa, as well as Davud Paşa, (Nakkaş?) Hasan Paşa, Yusuf Paşa, and Halil Paşa. Also present was the military judge of Rumeli Damad, Mevlânâ Muhammed, together with his predecessors Mevlânâ Es'adü'd-dîn, Yahya Efendi, Mevlânâ Mustafa, Mevlânâ 'Abdü'l-'Azîz,.and Taşköpri-zâde Mevlânâ Kemâlü'ddîn. The military judge of Anadolu, Ganîzâde Mevlânâ Muhammed, was similarly accompanied by his predecessors Bostanzâde Mevlânâ Muhammed and Ahîzâde Mevlânâ Hüseyin. They all arrived in Edirne on January 8 (Zilkade 16). See *Zübdetü 't-Tevârîh*, vol. 2, fols. 184b–186a.

52. *Zübdetü 't-Tevârîh*, vol. 2, fols. 189a–189b and 190a–190b: (1) At Florya, the first halting station after Davudpaşa, the Sultan's party stayed at the royal hunting lodge: *anda karârgâh-ı selâtîn ve nişîmen-i şikârgâh-ı havâkîn olan bağçe-i pür-behce kasr-ı 'âlîsinde nüzûl buyurdı. Ve ol gice anda havâss-ı mukarrebîn ve nedîmân-ı edeb-âyîn ile hakânî sohbet ve gicenin bir bahşi geçince müfâveza ve müsâhabet idüb*; (2) at Büyükçekmece, they stayed in a convenient house: *serîr-i saltanat-masîr üzre ârâm ve ol dâr u diyârı dîdâr-sa'âdet-âsârı ile şâdgâm eyledi.*

53. In their first stop at Florya, past Küçükçekmece, Ahmed I was keen to perform his prayers: *Zübdetü't-Tevârîh*, vol. 2, fols. 188b–189a.

54. Allsen, *Royal Hunt*, pp. 196–97.

55. Allsen, *Royal Hunt*, pp. 196–97.

56. Allsen, *Royal Hunt*, pp. 196–97.

57. *Zübdetü't-Tevârîh*, vol. 2, fol. 204b.

58. Various hawk species that are mentioned are *sunkur*, *şahin* or *balaban*.

59. *Zübdetü't-Tevârîh*, vol. 2, fols. 203b–204a: *hergün bir sebzezârı şikâr ve ahyânen taraf-ı nehârda bir kûşe vü kenârı ... sürgün şikârını arzû ve meyl-i sayd-ı hargûş (204a) ve rûbâh u âhû eylemegin, bostancıbaşı kullarına bu vechile emr-i 'âlî-kadr sâdır oldu ki, mahmiye-i Edrene havâlisinde olan şikârgâhlardan saydı çok ve vühûş-i behiminin hadd ü pâyânı yok bir mahalli taharrî itdikten sonra hidmetinde olan bostancılar ve kadîm-i eyyâm ve ezmân-ı selâtîn-i 'ızâmdan bu mekûle şikârlarda istihdâm ve bunun emsâli kârlarda kıyâm üzre olıgelen reayâdan bir nice karye ehâlîsi ile üç gün mukaddem varub, etrâf ü cevânibinden bir kaç günlük mesâfe-i ihâta vü zabt ve medâhil ü mehâricini sedd ü rabt ba'dehû ol kadar mesâfe içinde âremîde olan vühûş ü cânverânı manzar-ı pâdişâhî ve mahall-ı nazar-ı şehinşâhî olacak yere sevk tarîki ile remîde idüb.*

60. *Zübdetü't-Tevârîh*, vol. 2, fol. 205a: *ol şikârgâhın etrâf u cevânibin tutub kûh ü hâmûn ve ol mîşezâr-ı bî-çend ü çün hılâlinde sükûn iden vühûşı çi rûbâh ve çi har-gûş ve çi âhû ve çi gürg-i pür-hûrûşı sürüb, ol sahrâları ince elekten süzüb.*

61. *Zübdetü't-Tevârîh*, vol. 2, fol. 205b.

62. *Zübdetü't-Tevârîh*, vol. 2, fol. 206a.

63. *Zübdetü't-Tevârîh*, vol. 2, fol. 207a.

64. Compare with: Ebba Koch, *Dara-Shikoh Shooting Nilgais: Hunt and Landscape in Mughal Painting*, Occasional Papers (Washington: Freer Gallery of Art, 1998).

65. *Zübdetü't-Tevârîh*, vol. 2, fol. 208b.

66. *Zübdetü't-Tevârîh*, vol. 2, fol. 209a: *Çâşni ve lezzeti vasf olunsa nebât-ı hamevînin kadr-i pest ü hiç ve ehl-i mezâk huzûrunda zikr olunsa, cevâbı ol var ikem "şekerin ez, suyun iç" olur. Keyfiyyet-i hiffeti kemmiyet-i kesretini toyurmaz ve kemâl-i hâzimiyyeti kenârında ekl-i ta'am edeni asla toyurmaz.* Even the most reliable dictionaries do not yield any information on *nebât-ı hamavî*. The other references that I was able to find are in Evliyâ Çelebi. It appears as *Hamavî katr-ı nebât/ Ham[e]vî kandü'n-nebât* (vol. 1, pp. 278, 289, 360; vol. 2, pp. 206, 171, 190; vol. 3, p. 142; vol. 4, pp. 76, 159, 172;

vol. 10, p. 250); *katr-ı nebât-ı Hamavî* (vol. 1, p. 289; vol. 2, pp. 206, 171; vol. 3, p. 142; vol. 4, p. 159; vol. 5, pp. 125, 313; vol. 7, p. 110; vol. 8, pp. 45, 294; vol. 9, pp. 59, 96; vol. 10, p. 179), and *kand-i nebât-ı Ham[e]vî/kand-i nebât-ı Ham[e]viyyât* (vol. 1, pp. 278, 289, 360; vol. 2, pp. 206, 171, 190; vol. 3, p. 142; vol.4, pp. 76, 159, 172; vol. 10, p. 250): *Evliyâ Çelebi Seyahatnamesi. Topkapı Sarayı Kütüphanesi Bağdat 308 Numaralı Yazmanın Transkripsiyonu-Dizini. 1-10 kitap, ed.* O. Ş. Gökyay, Yücel Dağlı, Seyit Ali Kahraman, and Robert Dankoff (İstanbul: Yapı Kredi Yayınları, 1996–2007). See also: Robert Dankoff, *Evliya Çelebi in Bitlis 1655–1656: Relevant Section of the Seyahatname 1655–56* [Leiden: Brill, 1999], p. 310 [fol. 278b]). Still, *nebât-ı hamavî* can be identified as some kind of sugar from Hama, a town near Aleppo. (Syria had some of the best sugar cane reserves in the Middle Ages.) It appears to have consisted of large crystals of pure sugar that were given to people needing a jolt of energy. Apparently, this special sugar from Hama also had excellent digestive properties. Crystallized sugar is regularly listed in the daily or monthy kitchen allocations of the royal family and high-ranking dignitaries, and it was also used as an ingredient in traditional remedies for coughs and colds. Hence it seems to fall somewhere between a placebo and a homeopathic cure. It is a reminder of a time when sugar was a luxury and was accorded miraculous qualities. *Nebât-ı hamavî* was considerably more expensive than other kinds of sugar. See Ömer Lütfi Barkan, "İstanbul Saraylarına Ait Muhasebe Defterleri," *Belgeler* IX/13 (1979): p. 90.

67. *Zübdetü't-Tevârîh*, vol. 2, fol. 210a.

68. Felicity Heal, "Food Gifts, the Household and the Politics of Exchange in Early Modern England," *Past and Present* 199, (May 2008): pp. 41–70.

69. Gelibolulu Âli gives priority to venison. "Second in order," he says, "are the cranes, geese, pheasants, partridges that fly like the *hümâ* bird—all the foods of manifest superiority belonging to the category of game birds." Thirdly, he lists the beasts and quadrupeds the eating of some of which is permitted, and "whose fresh meat yields a delicious taste unequalled anywhere." Included are gazelles and hares. Fourthly, he lists fish, the consuming of which he finds manifestly delectable. (It should be noted that Gelibolu alludes to attractive young males as also game.) Sixteenth-century palace account books studied by Barkan, as well as Evliya's numerous references to hunting parties and banquets, help to identify the game animals consumed by the Ottoman elite in the environs of İstanbul: Ömer Lütfi Barkan, "İstanbul Saraylarına Ait Muhasebe Defterleri," *Belgeler* IX/13, (1979), pp. 1–380; *Evliya Çelebi Seyahatnamesi. Topkapı Sarayı Bağdad 304 Yazmasının Transkripsiyonu-Dizini* I, ed. Orhan Şaik Gökyay (İstanbul: Yapı Kredi Yayınları, 1996), pp. 194, 196, 208, 254. In Europe, it is venison that also appears most regularly in literature about food giving. We are told that "even the physicians, who were uneasy

that the timorous nature of the deer might infect its eaters, often swallowed their dietary doubts when faced with the food of lords. Andrew Boorde, a doctor, confessed somewhat hesitantly to an affection for venison, adding 'I am sure it is a lordes dysshe, and I am sure it is good for an Englysshe man, for it doth animate hym to be as he is; whiche is stronge and hardye'" (Andrew Boorde, *The fyrst boke of the introduction of knowledge made by Andrew Borde, of physycke doctor. A compendyous regyment; or, A dyetary of helth made in Mountpyllier*, ed. Frederic James Furnivall, Extra Series [London: published for the Early English Text Society, 1870], pp. 274–75), after Heal, "Food Gifts," p. 57. Heal also notes the contrast here with the pattern revealed for a slightly earlier period in Chris Woolgar's study of three East Anglian households of the fourteenth century. No gifts of venison were recorded, indeed it is not mentioned in any of the accounts, and, beyond the ubiquitous capons, the most common offerings were swans and fish, including salted herring (Chris Woolgar, "Diet and Consumption in Gentry and Noble Households: A Case Study from around the Wash," in *Rulers and Ruled in Late Medieval England: Essays Presented to Gerald Harriss*, ed. Rowena E. Archer and Simon Walker [London: Hambledon Press, 1995], pp. 17–32).

70. *Zübdetü't-Tevârîh*, vol. 2, fol. 210a.

71. *Zübdetü't-Tevârîh*, vol. 2, fols. 210b–211a.

72. *Zübdetü't-Tevârîh*, vol. 2, fol. 210a: *âş-pezân-ı sebük-dest ve helvaciyân-ı şeker-şikest ahşâmdan tabh u ihzâr ve tertîbinde san'atlar ızhâr itdikleri nefâis-i et'ime ve hulviyyât-ı nefîse-i mütenevvi a-yı nazar-ı iksîr nazîrlerine getürilüb.*

73. *Zübdetü't-Tevârîh*, vol. 2, fols. 210a–210b: *çün kânûn-ı hümâyûn-ı Osmânî ve töre-i meymûn-ı sultânî bu vech üzredir ki, hazret-i padişâh-ı 'âlî-câh içün sarây-ı 'âmir-i sultânîden hâne-i hâss-ı hâkânîde veya büyük yimekliklerde (210b) bast-ı mâide-i ta'âm ve ferş-i süfre-i mahz-ı in'âm olunsa, ser-i kileri-yân ve ser-kâr-ı gıdâ-yı hazret-i hüdâvendigâr olan ağa kulları ol hidmete mütesaddî ve hazret-i pâdişâh-ı saltanat-penâh müşarûnileyh elinden müte'aşşî ve mütegaddî olurlar. Ve mûmâileyh hâzır olmaduğı mevâtında sofra-ı ta'âm ve mâide-i berekât-encâmı silâhdarlık hıdmetine kıyâm ve ol hıdmet-i şerîfe makâmında devâm üzre olan bende-i hâss ve mukarrib-i bâ-ihlâs kulları bast ve evâni-i zehebiyye vaz' u ref'i maslahatını rabt ider.*

74. For the assiduous piety of the sultan: Artan, "A Book of Kings," pp. 299–330.

75. *Zübdetü't-Tevârîh*, vol. 2, fol. 212a.

76. *Zübdetü't-Tevârîh*, vol. 2, fol. 212b.

77. *Zübdetü't-Tevârîh*, vol. 2, fols. 213a and 214a.

78. *Zübdetü't-Tevârîh*, vol. 2, fol. 213b.

79. *Zübdetü 't-Tevârîh*, vol. 2, fol. 214a.

80. *Zübdetü 't-Tevârîh*, vol. 2, fol. 213a: *vüzerâ ve kuzât-ı 'asker meclis-i ârâya dahî gelüb, sayd-gâhdan pâdişâh-ı 'âlem-penâh hazretlerinin manzarı olmayan birer mahallden temâşâ ve ol me 'dübe-i 'azîme tenâvülinde müşâreket-i ehillâ itmek içün da 'vet ve vezîr-i a 'zam tarafından işâret olunub.*

81. *Zübdetü 't-Tevârîh*, vol. 2, fol. 214a.

82. *Zübdetü 't-Tevârîh*, vol. 2, fol. 215a: *âlât-ı tabh-ı ni 'am ve esbâb-ı 'îş-i safâ müdgam ile tabbâhân-ı tîz-kâr ve helvâ-pezân-ı sebük-kirdârı ol cây-ı ma 'hûd ve mahall-i mev 'ûde gönderüb, hassâ-ı pâdişâhî olan mâide-i şehen-şâhî içün nefâis-i et 'ime-i lezîze ve sanâif-i halâvat ve eşribe-i nefîse ihzârın sipâriş itdiklerinden .*

83. *Zübdetü 't-Tevârîh*, vol. 2, fol. 215a: *çeşm-i harîsân ve zahâmet-i vüs 'atde mi 'de-i gedâ-çeşmân gibi olan müte 'addid kazganlar içinde pilâv ü zerde ve nazîr u mislin nâ-dîde vü nâ-horde oldukları kalye vü nehyî-i perverde tabhın işâret eylediler.*

84. It is wrong to take *kalye* as a vegetarian dish. For nearly two dozen recipes, see: Muhammed bin Mahmud Şirvani, *15. Yüzyıl Osmanlı Mutfağı. Muhammed bin Mahmûd Şirvanî*, ed. Mustafa Argunşah and Müjgan Çakır (İstanbul: Gökkubbe Yayınları, 2005), pp. 75–89.

85. *Zübdetü 't-Tevârîh*, vol. 2, fol. 217b: *zer ü sîm ile çeşm-i kâni 'veş memlû ve nukra-ı mazrûb ve ibrîz-i meskûk-ı keder meslûb ile misâl-i derûn-ı ganiyyü 'l-kalbi dâmen-keş toptolu kîsehâ-yı müte 'addid ve hemyânhâ-yı müteceddide ile zînet ve nazîr-i esdâf-ı dürr, zer ü sîm ile pür-tabakhâ-yı sîm ve rakîbehâ-yı 'azîmden mâ 'adâ mücevher matharalar ve murassa 'gülâbdan ve maşrabalar tertîbi ile misâl-i erîke-i cennet olmuş.*

86. *Zübdetü 't-Tevârîh*, vol. 2, fol. 218a: *et 'ime-i hoş-güvâr ve ağdiye-i nefâset-medâr ile a 'dâd-ı nücûm-ı âsmânı tabakhâ-yı lâhûr u mertabâni ve sahanhâ-yı çînî-i zümürred-sânî çekilüb.*

87. *Zübdetü 't-Tevârîh*, vol. 2, fol. 218b.

88. *Zübdetü 't-Tevârîh*, vol. 2, fol. 218b.

89. The tent reserved for the sultan is called *hayme* or *bâlâ-yı püştede nasb olunan hargâh-ı şâhî* (*Zübdetü 't-Tevârîh*, vol. 2, fol. 220a).

90. *Zübdetü 't-Tevârîh*, vol. 2, fols. 219b–221a. For another pictorial weather report: *Zübdetü 't-Tevârîh*, vol. 1, fol. 150a.

91. *Zübdetü 't-Tevârîh*, vol. 2, fols. 221b–223b.

92. *Zübdetü 't-Tevârîh*, vol. 2, fols. 223b–224b.

93. As with most low-fat game animals, modern cookbooks require venison to be cooked very slowly (less than 300 degrees) to keep from drying out. While

vegetables and fruits help to keep moisture in, a nineteenth-century Ottoman cookbook suggests that after being marinated in onion juice and salt, large chunks of deer, roe deer, and chamois meat should be skewed alternatingly with fatty ram meat and moisturized with fatty bouillon while on the fire (Ayşe Fahriye, *Ev Kadını*, tr. Leman Erdemli and Zeynep Vanlı [İstanbul: Ofset Yapımevi, 2002], p. 43; original Ottoman edition: Dersaadet: Arif Efendi Matbaası, 1323 [1905/6]).

94. *Zübdetü't-Tevârîh*, vol. 2, fol. 223b.

95. The word *miskiyye* crops up yet again, suggesting a kind of sweet drink prepared from the musk glands or any other parts of *Viverridae* family, comprising civets, mongooses, and meerkats.

96. *Zübdetü't-Tevârîh*, vol. 2, fols. 223b–224b: *.vezîr-ı a'zam ... bendeleri tertîbinde tekellüf ve tabh u tehzîbinde telattuf eyledügi nefâis-i et'ime-i hoş-güvâr ve sanâif-i ağdiye-i çâşnidâr ki, tabbâhân-ı pâkîze-dest ve âş-pezân-ı çâşnîbest, tamâm-ı san'at ve kemâl-i hikmet ile nâr-ı leyyine ve âteş-i hâdîye üzre tabh idüb, her birine misk ü 'anber ta'biye ve 'akâkîr-i mu'teber ile terbiye itmegin revâyih-i tayyibeleri dimâğ-ı rûhânîyâni ta'tîr ü tervîh ve fevâyih-i miskiyye-i zekiyyeleri meşâm-ı mele-i a'lâyı tetyîb ve sudur-ı nûrânîyânı tefrîh u teşrîh ider idi. Sahanhâ-yı zerrîn ve tabakhâ-yı sîmîn içine mevzû' ve ekvâb-ı merfû'a (224a) misâl-i meclis-i 'âlî-i şâhîye merfû olub nazar-ı iksîr eserlerinde mebsûta olan mâide-i zer-kûb ve sofra-i berekât-ı mashûbe nihâde ve ser-pûş-ı zerrîneleri küşâde olıcak, her bir ta'âm-ı lâtîfeden hazların musîb ve her kısım gıdâ-yı nefis ü şerîfden âhiz-i nâsib oldılar. Ve çün sadru'l-vüzera bendeleri hayme-i zer-kâr ve ol har-gâh-ı pür-kârdan verâ-i perde bir mahallde vâkıf u hâzır ve ol metâ'im-i lezîzenin keyfıyyet-i vaz'ına bir kûşeden nâzır idügin hazret-i pâdişâh-ı bâ-vakâr ihsâs u istiş'âr eylemiş idi. Kasd-ı ta'zîm ve irâde-i tekrîm ile mâide-i pür-'âideden anlara hıssa ve pes horde-i şeref-bürde-i bâ-fâideden behre irsâli ile kadrini i'lâ ve şe'nini tenvîh ile ref'-i mertebe-i 'ulyâ eylediler ve çün emr-i ta'âm itmâm (224b) ve münâvele-i eşribe-i miskiyyetü'l-hıtâm ikmâl olunub i'mâl-i âfitâbe vü ibrîk ve isti'mâl-i gülâb ü 'anber ile meşâmlar tenşîk olundı. Ol sofra-ı pür behreden nevâlehor ve zelle-ber olan nüdemâ istîfâ-i kadr-ı iştihâ eyleyecek her biri ayağ üzre gelüb devâm-ı devletlerine du'â ve cenâb-ı hazretlerine senâ idüb.*

97. *Zübdetü't-Tevârîh* vol. 2, fols. 227b–229a.

98. For *Tuhfetü'l-mülûk ve's-selatin* see: TülayArtan, "A Book of Kings." For the original: Topkapı Palace Museum Library H. 415; 385 mm by 250mm; 253 pages; 164 miniatures and 2 illuminated pages. See also: Fehmi Edhem Karatay, *Topkapı Sarayı Müzesi Kütüphanesi Türkçe Yazmalar Kataloğu* (İstanbul: TSM Yayınları, 1961), vol. 1, pp. 574–75. For other Ottoman hunting treatises, see: Halûk Aydın, "Ebû Bekr İbnü'l-Hacî Mustafa Kızılhisârî'nin

Avcılıkla İlgili Bir Eseri: Hidâyetü's Sayyâd," in *Av ve Avcılık Kitabı*, ed. Emine Gürsoy-Naskali and Hilal Oytun Altun (İstanbul: Kitabevi Yayınları, 2008), pp. 653–96; and Fahrettin Coşkuner and Sait Okumuş, "Av ve Avcılığa Dair XV. Yüzyılda Yazılmış Bir Av Risâlesi: Sayd-nâme," in *Av ve Avcılık Kitabı*, ed. Emine Gürsoy-Naskali and Hilal Oytun Altun (İstanbul: Kitabevi Yayınları, 2008), pp. 697–707.

99. Recently, Marc Baer, too, has underlined that hunting demonstrated the Ottoman sultans' (in particular, Mehmed IV's) bravery and courage, hence manliness (*merdânelik*), and was a training for warfare. Baer is mistaken, however, in saying that in the opinion of the chroniclers he studies there was nothing pathological about hunting, and that the perception of hunting as a frivolous activity is a modern construction. See: Marc D. Baer, *Honoured by the Glory of Islam. Conversion and Conquest in Ottoman Europe* (Oxford: Oxford University Press, 2008), pp. 180–81. Compare with: *The Ottoman Gentleman of the Sixteenth Century*, p. 38; and Tülay Artan, "A Book of Kings."

100. For the return trip: *Zübdetü't-Tevârîh*, vol. 2, fols. 229b–247a.

101. For the princes: *Zübdetü't-Tevârîh*, vol. 2, fol. 310a.

102. *Zübdetü't-Tevârîh*, vol. 2, fols. 301b–303a.

103. *Zübdetü't-Tevârîh*, vol. 2, fols. 303b–309a.

104. *Zübdetü't-Tevârîh*, vol. 2, fol. 305a.

105. *Zübdetü't-Tevârîh*, vol. 2, fols. 309b–312a. Compare with a banquet in İstanbul: *Zübdetü't-Tevârîh*, vol. 2, fols. 320b–321a.

106. *Zübdetü't-Tevârîh*, vol. 2, fols. 326b–336a.

107. *Zübdetü't-Tevârîh*, vol. 2, fol. 332b: *vakt-i câşt ve ta'âm-ı gıdâ içün zamân-ı fürû-dâşt olmağın…(333a)…ta'âm-ı kerem ve nân-ı sepîd-nerm hâzır olmak içün te'lîf olunan matbah-ı revândan pişgâh-ı sultânîye hân-ı firâvân çekilüb, hazret-i şâh-ı nâmdâr ol et'ime-i lezîze-i hôş-güvârdan güvârdan istîfâ-i merâm ve ahz-i murâd u kâm itdikten sonra.* Later, Mustafa Sâfî eulogizes this expedition with a *kasîde* and refers to this banquet. *Zübdetü't-Tevârîh*, vol. 2, fol. 340a:

Kıldı nüzûl haymeye şâh-ı cihân o dem
Geldi miyâne et'ime-i hôb-ı hoş-güvâr

Etrâf-ı meclise dikilüb turdı sad-nedîm
Her biri bezle kûy-ı sahun-senc ü nükte-bâr

Destûr oldı söylediler çok letâifı
Güldi açıldı gül gibi ol gonca-i bahâr

Çünkim ta'âm emri tamâm oldı hamd idüb
Oldı süvâr-ı esb-i sebük-rev o şehsüvâr

108. *Zübdetü't-Tevârîh*, vol. 2, fol. 345a.

109. *Zübdetü't-Tevârîh*, vol. 2, fols. 338a–360b. For a banquet at Çömlek:
Zübdetü't-Tevârîh, vol. 2, fols. 352b:

O şâhın makdemi kevn-i subh u şâma
İdeler sa'y-ı ihzâr-ı ta'âma

İdeler tabh-ı envâ'-ı nefâis
Ki, idrâk idemiye fikr-i kâyis

Pîşe envâ'-ı hulviyât-ı ra'nâ
Lühûm-ı berre vü mürg-i murabbâ

Bunu vasf eylesem ta'bîre gelmez
Ki, zevkidir belî takrîre gelmez

Ve ger hem güfte bûdeş sâhib-i şâh
Ki, ez-behr-i havâss u 'âmme-i râh

Pezed yekpâre çendân gûsfendî
Ki, yâbed behre zû sad müstemendî

Bi kazgan-ı ferâhî çendî hem âş
Pilâv u zerde ni mencû vü ni mâş

Şüd puhte berây-i merdüm-i 'âm
Hôrend ü hoş berend ân kavm-i nâ kâm

110. Respectively: *Zübdetü't-Tevârîh*, vol. 2, fols. 364a–365a and 353b–354a.

111. *Zübdetü't-Tevârîh'i*, vol. 2, fol. 215a.

112. A modern translation, "fruits cooked in sherbet, marmalade," is provided by Stefanos Yerasimos, *Sultan Sofraları: 15. ve 16. Yüzyılda Osmanlı Saray Mutfağı* (İstanbul: Yapı ve Kredi Yayınları, 2002), p. 145.

113. There is no mention of *nehy-i perverde* in the translation by Ahmed Cavid (d. 1803) of Mevlânâ Ebû İshak Hallâcı Şirâzî (d. 1423 or 1427), *Tercüme-i Kenzü'l-İştihâ: 15. Yüzyıldan Bir Mutfak Sözlüğü*, ed. Seyit Ali Kahraman and Priscilla Mary Işın (İstanbul: Kitap Yayınevi, 2006). In the section "*Terkib-i tuffahiyye ve seferceliyye*," *perverde* is referred as a cooking process: *ol şeker*

içinde perverde pişüre. In modern recipes, the equivalent might be boiling fruits or dried fruits until they reach a certain viscosity. Then fresh butter and walnuts would be added.

114. Tabîb İbn-i Şerîf, *Yâdigâr: 15. Yüzyıl Türkçe Tıb Kitabı. Yadigâr-ı İbn-i Şerîf,* ed. M. Yahya Okutan, Doğan Koçer and Mecit Yıldız (İstanbul: Yerküre Yayınları, 2004), p. 248: *tâze koruk suyun üzerine koyub havân içinde sahk idüb adetce perverde idüb.* In the dictionary section of *Yâdigâr,* there is another reference to *perverde* which, in this case, is marinated garlic, *perverde-i sevm:* pp. 442 and 446 (fol. 304b).

115. Semih Tezcan, *Bir Ziyafet Defteri* (İstanbul: Simurg Yayınları, 1998), p. 9 (fol. 43b).

116. Tezcan, *Bir Ziyafet Defteri,* p. 13 (fol. 44b), p. 15 (fol. 45a).

117. Şirvani, *15. Yüzyıl Osmanlı Mutfağı.*

118. For recipes of *tuffahiye* and *seferceliye:* Şirvani, *15. Yüzyıl Osmanlı Mutfağı,* pp. 59 and 242 (fols. 11a–11b and 127b–128b). See also the new translation of Muhammad b. Al-Hasan b. Muhammad b. Al-Karîm, the scribe of Baghdad, *A Baghdad Cookery Book: The Book of Dishes (Kitâb al-Tabîkh)* tr. Charles Perry (Trowbridge: Cromwell Press, 2005), pp. 34–35 and 55–56. While *tuffahiyya* is listed under "sour dishes and their varieties," *safarjaliyya* is listed among "fried and dry dishes."

119. For a *kabak kalye* recipe, cooked in unriped grape juice and sweetened with grape juice (if in season; if not, with honey or sugar): M. Nejat Sefercioğlu, *Türk Yemekleri: XVIII. Yüzyıla Ait Bir Yemek Risâlesi* (Ankara: Kültür ve Turizm Bakanlığı, 1985), p. 59.

120. Feyzi Halıcı, *Ali Eşref Dede'nin Yemek Risalesi* (Ankara: Atatürk Kültür Merkezi Yayınları, 1992).

121. I am grateful to Ms. Nacmieh Batmanglij who has kindly brought this possibility to my attention (Montreal, November 20, 2007). As Batmanglij notes, Muslims who wished to consume alcohol had a variety of excuses: wine was being drunk as a medicine; it was alleged that the Koran only forbade over-indulgence in wine; the ban applied only to wine and not to arak, beer, or fermented mare's milk. See her recipes with wine: Nacmieh Batmanlij, *From Persia to Napa. Wine at the Persian Table* (Washington, DC: Mage Publications, 2006).

122. *Zübdetü't-Tevârîh,* vol. 2, fol. 358b.

123. Elif Ayla, *Şerbet ve Hoşaf: Hatıralarda Kalan Yudum Yudum Lezzetler* (İstanbul: Hayy Yayınları, 2009). The following succinct summary is from Julliette Rossant, "The World's First Soft Drink," *Saudi Aramco World* 56/5 (September–October 2005): pp. 36–39: "One variant, Arabic *sharbah* (essentially

"a drink"), has given us Turkish *şerbet* (and Persian and Hindi *sharbat*) and our [Western] sherbet. Another, *shurb* (literally "a drinking"), followed trading ships back west with Portuguese *xarope*, giving Medieval Latin *sirupus* and our own rather Greek-looking *syrup*. More recently, *sharaab* came west from India and by 1867 had entered such dictionaries as Smith's *Sailor's Wordbook*, which lists "Shrab, a vile drugged drink prepared for seamen who frequent the filthy purlieus of Calcutta. The spelling in the American colonies crystallized as shrub."

124. For a recent study on visual narratives with the theme of wine–drinking: Meera Khane, "The Wine-Cup in Mughal Court Culture. From Hedonism to Kingship," *The Medieval History Journal* 8 (2005): pp. 143–188.

125. Batmanlij, *From Persia to Napa*, 45. Firdausi's *Shahname* abounds in hunting and drinking scenes. For more examples: Ehsan Yarshater, "The Theme of Wine-Drinking and the Concept of the Beloved in Early Persian Poetry," *Studia Islamica* 13 (1960): pp. 43–53.

126. *Halal*: goat, sheep, cattle, buffalo, buck, fish, camel, gazelle, onager, rabbit, fowls, ducks, pigeon, sparrow, partridge, crane, locusts, bustard, owl, swift, giraffe, magpie, quail, lark, starling, sand grouse, nightingale, ostrich, peacock, goose, turtle dove, stag, swan, dolphin, shark. *Haram*: insects, snake, lizard, gecko, mice, rats, hedgehog, jerboa, weasel, frog, lion, wolf, jackal, leopard, tiger, lynx, cheetah, panther, fox, cat, squirrel, fennel, sable, bear, monkey, ape, elephant, dog, falcon, hawk, saker, kite, eagle, vulture, bat, tortoise, crocodile, mongoose, ferret, raven. Note, incidentally, that all the weasels, ferrets, and mongooses of the *Viverridae* (source of *miskiyye*) are classified as *haram*. See Gelibolulu Âli on game animals the eating of which were permitted: *The Ottoman Gentleman of the Sixteenth Century*, pp. 38–40. See also: Yusuf Ziya Keskin, "Hadislere Göre Avlanma Kuralları," in *Av ve Avcılık Kitabı*, ed. Emine Gürsoy-Naskali and Hilal Oytun Altun (İstanbul: Kitabevi Yayınları, 2008), pp. 497–514.

127. *Zübdetü't-Tevârîh*, vol. 2, fol. 223b.

128. Elisabeth Borromeo, "The Ottomans and Hunting According to Julien Bordier's Travelogue," in *Animals and People in the Ottoman Empire*, ed. Suraiya Faroqhi (Istanbul: Eren Yayınları, forthcoming), pp. 215–31. I am grateful to my colleague for allowing me to consult her manuscript. Julien Bordier, mss.cit, fol. 186v: "Sy ce prend quelque bestes fauve elles distribuée aux esclaves chretiens car les Turcs ne mangent de venaison que rarement principallement des animaux quy nonts esté saigné que de main d'hommes tenent en cela du judaisme." Sonnini, too, makes the same point at the end of the eighteenth century, when the royal hunt was abandoned for good: C. S. Sonnini, *Voyage en Grèce et Turquie*, 2 vols. (Paris : Buisson, 1891), vol 2,

p. 163: "La seule précaution qu'ils prennent, lorsqu'ils ont abattu une pièce de gibier, est de se hater de la saigner au cou, afin de ne point contrevenir à une autre loi qui leur defend de faire usage de la chair d'un animal qui n'auroit pas été saigné, et cette precaution nuit à la saveur du gibier."

129. Julien Bordier, mss.cit, fol. 495r.: "Le gibier nest surbatu comme il est en Crestienne, les turcs nestant eusitez à la chasse de l'Arquebuse, qui est ce qui espouvante le plus le gibier." If it happened that the Turks (only *acemioğlan*s and janissaries, Bordier writes) went shooting, it was because they had seen the (French) ambassador and his suite hunt. Julien Bordier, mss.cit, fol. 495v: "Il est bien vray que quelque Janissaire du pays à nostre imitation sen vouloit escrimer sur le lac (Küçükçekmece) où ne sentendoit qu'arquebusade de bout à autre, mais pour ester de deux grand lieu de long, & une du large, le gibier avoit beau sesgayer & les gibayeurs aussy. "

130. Mehmet Ertuğrul Düzdağ, *Şeyhülislam Ebussud Efendi Fetvaları Işığında 16. Asır Türk Hayatı* (İstanbul: Enderun Kitabevi, 1983), p. 190.

131. François Viré, "Jurisprudence en matière de gibier tué à plomb. *Risâla tuhfat al-hawass fî hill sayd bunduq al-rasâs,*" *Bulletin d'études orientales* 30 (1978): pp. 289–305.

132. From a *fatwa* point of view, hunting for pleasure is permissible if one does not become unmindful of his obligations, for example, performing the *namaz*, which is generally among the consequences of hunting. The Prophet is accepted to have said: "Whosoever follows an animal of the hunt, (generally) becomes unmindful." Life is extremely short and cannot be wasted on futilities, i.e., activities that are neither a worldly need nor of any benefit in the hereafter. It is best to abstain. This is an all-encompassing principle.

133. Almond, *Medieval Hunting*, p. 20, and especially chapter 3.

134. Almond, *Medieval Hunting*, p. 85.

135. All this information comes from Sonja Freifrau von Müffling, "Cooking with Game," in *Game and Hunting*, ed. Kurt G. Blüchel (Cologne: Könemann, 1977), pp. 586–613.

136. For formal banquet scenes: (1) Lala Mustafa Paşa throwing a banquet for the high officials at İznikmid during the Eastern campaign of 1578–80: *Nusretnâme*, TSM H. 1365 (1584), fol. 34b; (2) Ferhat Paşa giving a banquet in honour of Prince Haydar in Erzurum during the 1588 eastern campaign: *Kitâb-ı Gencine-i Feth-i Gence*, TSM R. 1296 (1590), fol. 48b; and (3) the sultan's banquet at the Hippodrome during the 1582 circumcision festivities for his son Mehmed (the future Mehmed III): *Surnâme-i Hümâyûn*, TSM H. 1344 (1587), fols. 74b–75a.

137. Vienna, Österreische National Bibliothek, Codex Mixtus 313, fol. 28b. The

muraqqa album was made in Istanbul in 980 AH/1572–73 AD): Aimée E. Froom, "Collecting Tastes: A Muraqqa' for Sultan Murad III," *Electronic Journal of Oriental Studies* 4 (2001).

138. Aimée E. Froom, "A Muraqqa' for the Ottoman Sultan Murad III (r. 1574–1595): ÖsterreichischeNationalbibliothek, Codex Mixtus 313" (PhD. diss., Institute of Fine Arts, NY, 2001), p. 437; Aimée E. Froom, "Adorned Like a Rose: the Persian Connection in the *Muraqqa* for the Ottoman Sultan Murad III (Austrian National Library, Cod. Mixt. 313)," *Artibus Asiae* 66/2 (2006): pp. 137–54.

139. Emmy Wellesz, "Die Miniaturen im Album Murad III," *Wiener Beitrage Zur Kunst und Kulturgeschichte Asiens 10* (1936): pp. 55–67; G. M. Meredith-Owens, *Turkish Miniatures* (London: British Museum Publications, 1963), pl. VIII; Rachel Milstein, *Miniature Painting in Ottoman Baghdad* (Costa Mesa CA: Mazda Publications, 1990), fig.42. An eighteenth-century miniature showing ladies picnicking along the Bosphorus also depicts the attendants roasting meat on a spit: Tülay Artan, "Boğaziçi'nin Çehresini Değiştiren Soylu Kadınlar ve Sultanefendi Sarayları," *İstanbul Dergisi* 3 (1992): pp. 109–18.

140. *Ahmed I Album*, Topkapı Palace Library B. 408, fols. 14a, 19a.

141. İstanbul University Library T. 6624, fol. 100b. Compare also with a slightly earlier copy of the *Tercüme-i Miftâh Cifrü'l-Câmî*: Topkapı Palace Library B. 373 (1597–98), fol. 243b.

142. See fols. 232v, a garden party with a lady and four attendants; 232r, a king (in a garden kiosk?) with a falcon, a guest, and three attendants; 241v, a garden party, with a dancer, a *ney* player, a *çeng* player, and a *def* player; 241r, a garden party, with two *def* players, an *ud* player, and a *zil* player; 245v, a king with a guest and two attendants; 245r, a lady with three attendants; 249v, a lady (in a garden kiosk) with five attendants; 249r, a king in a kiosk with a guest and three armed attendants; 250v, a lady in a garden with four attendants; 250r, a king in a garden with a guest and three armed attendants; 251v, a king in a kiosk with a falcon, receiving a guest and attended by two armed attendants; 251r, a king in a garden with a falcon, receiving a guest and attended by three armed attendants; 252v, a lady in a garden with four attendants; and 252r, a king in a garden with a falcon, receiving a guest in the presence of three armed attendants.

143. Tülay Artan, "Art and Architecture," in *The Cambridge History of Turkey*, vol. III, *The Later Ottoman Empire, 1603–1839*, ed. Suraiya Faroqhi (Cambridge: Cambridge University Press, 2006), pp. 408–80.

144. It should also be noted that in the early seventeenth-century Ottoman minitures to which we have been referring, there would always be a person of status seated to the right of the throne, recalling Asaf ibn Barkhiya, the wise and the

learned vizier of Solomon. This goes back to a very common model in Islamic painting: the depictions of Solomon and Bılqıs, the Queen of Sheba, enthroned outdoors, in "nature," and surrounded by animals, birds, and supernatural creatures.

145. Serpil Bağcı, "From Translated Word to Translated Image: The Illustrated Şehnâme-i Türkî Copies," *Muqarnas* 17 (2000): pp. 162–76.

146. Secondary literature on the Ottoman *sehnâma*s claims that the chain of continuity was broken during the term of Talikizâde. First, *Şehnâme-i Talikizâde* misses out the final years of Murad III's reign, 1593–95. Furthermore, what Talikizâde penned down for Mehmed III is rather a campaign book: *Fetihnâme-i Eğri*. With no illustrated history eulogizing the reign of Ahmed I located, it has been argued that the tradition was resumed by the *Şehnâme-i Nadirî*, narrating also just a single military expedition—Osman II's Hotin campaign in 1621–22. See: Christine Woodhead, "An Experiment in Official Historiography: The Post of Şehnameci in the Ottoman Empire," *Wiener Zeitschrift für die Kunde des Morgenlandes* 75 (1983): pp. 157–82

"Mr. Turkey Goes to Turkey," Or: How an Eighteenth-Century Dutch Diplomat Lunched at Topkapı Palace*

JOANITA VROOM

Introduction

Turkish cuisine is often considered as *haute cuisine*, i.e., a cuisine based on a highly developed courtly society and social competition. In this perspective it ranks among the Chinese, Indian and French cuisines.[1] Being influenced by Persian, Chinese, and Middle Eastern flavors, Turkish cuisine attained its height during the Ottoman period (ca. fifteenth–nineteenth centuries).

Nowadays, we know quite a lot about the culinary aspects of the Ottoman elite in this period because visitors from the West described the eating habits at the court in Istanbul. In fact, these foreigners often described the table customs at Topkapı Palace often in more detail than the residents, because as outsiders they were in a position to record what was 'peculiar' (to them) in the Ottoman etiquette and culinary conventions.[2]

* I would like to thank Amy Singer for initiating this publication and editing my article in it. For the preparation of this article I was awarded a Senior Research Fellowship at the Research Center for Anatolian Civilizations, Koç University, Istanbul, in the academic year 2006–2007. I am very grateful to the Center, to its director, Dr. Scott Redford, and to the other 2006–2007 Research Fellows for providing an inspiring and supportive environment. A shorter version of this article previously appeared in M. Caroll, D. M. Hadley and H. Willmott, eds., *Consuming Passions: Dining from Antiquity to the Eighteenth Century* (Stroud, Gloucestershire: Tempus Carroll, 2005), pp. 143–61, but unfortunately without any notes..

The aim of this article is to catch a glimpse of the wining and dining habits at the Ottoman court in Istanbul as seen through the eyes of such an outsider, the eighteenth-century ambassador of the Dutch Republic at the Porte, Cornelis Calkoen (1696–1764). In addition, it deals with the Ottoman rules of etiquette relating to eating and drinking, often derived from Islamic doctrine, and in a wider sense with the development of dining manners in the Ottoman Empire from the late fifteenth to the eighteenth centuries.

All this is approached from an archaeological perspective. Therefore, special emphasis is put on the material aspects of Turkish cuisine, in particular the kitchen utensils and dining equipment used in the imperial kitchens of Topkapı Palace in Istanbul. Here, Chinese porcelain, copper, and silverware as well as locally produced tin-glazed ceramics (such as Iznik and Kütahya wares) were stored in large quantities.

Imperial kitchen records and Ottoman miniatures give some idea of how these high-quality wares were used during sumptuous banquets. However, Iznik and Kütahya wares were not exclusively used at the sultan's table in Istanbul. Recent excavations in Greece and the Balkans have revealed that they were also known in the provinces of the Ottoman Empire.

Cornelis Calkoen Visits the Sultan

On Sunday, September, 14, 1727, the ambassador of the Dutch Republic, Cornelis Calkoen, had the honor of being received in audience at the Ottoman court by Sultan Ahmed III (r. 1703–30). Calkoen made an extensive description of this special visit to the sultan and his son-in-law, the grand vizier Damad İbrahim Pasha. This report is now in the State Archives in The Hague and will here be referred to as the "*Relaes*."[3]

Cornelis Calkoen was born on May 21, 1696, into a wealthy patrician's family from Amsterdam (Figure 1). The family name means in Dutch "Turkey," as in the name of the bird which is traditionally served during Thanksgiving, not as in the name of the country which rose from the debris of the Ottoman Empire.[4] Known as a friendly gentleman of enormous stature, he was ambassador of the Dutch Republic to the Porte in Constantinople from 1725 to 1743. Apparently, he owed this post to the efforts of a relative, Amsterdam's mayor Jan Six II (1668–1750), who belonged to the well-known Dutch Six family and who was a descendent of the more favorably known Jan Six I (1618–1700), also mayor of Amsterdam and in the seventeenth century a well-known friend of Rembrandt, who painted a famous portrait of him.[5] As a diplomat Cornelis Calkoen was not particularly successful, but his personality and stature seemed to appeal to the imagination of future generations. Long after his death in 1764 there still were many rumors told about him and his beautiful mistresses.

Among these the most legendary was Beyaz Gül, or "White Rose," a Circassian slave who remained in Istanbul after Calkoen was posted to Dresden. Her relation with Calkoen was depicted

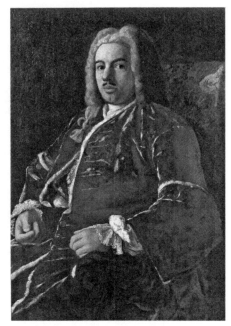

Figure 1. Portrait of the Dutch ambassador Cornelis Calkoen (1696-1764), by Jean-Baptiste Vanmour. Amsterdam, Rijksmuseum A 1996

allegorically on a tortoiseshell snuffbox, which is still in the possession of Calkoen's family, depicting the corpulent ambassador as a fat turkey and his mistress as the goddess Venus held on a chain by the god Amor in the background.[6] Apparently, when Calkoen left Beyaz Gül behind in Istanbul in 1744, she is said to have died from grief.[7] Eventually, all of Calkoen's love stories found a literary epitome in M. C. van Zeggelen's historical novel *Grand Seigneur*, which features Calkoen as the leading character.[8]

Cornelis Calkoen not only wrote a detailed report about his audience at the court of Sultan Ahmed III (r. 1703–30) to his principals (the Bureau of Levantine Trade in Amsterdam), he also wanted for himself a painted account of this important event. To that end he commissioned the French painter Jean-Baptiste Vanmour (1671–1737), who was noted for his realistic and truthful audience-pictures made for several French ambassadors and a Swedish diplomat in the early eighteenth century. In fact, Vanmour's work was becoming so famous among Constantinople's diplomatic circles that the increasing amount of orders forced him to found a "school" with assistants.[9]

Cornelis Calkoen's collection of "Turkish" paintings by Vanmour and his school is nowadays in the storage-rooms of the Rijksmuseum at Amsterdam. The Calkoen bequest numbers sixty-five oil paintings, most of

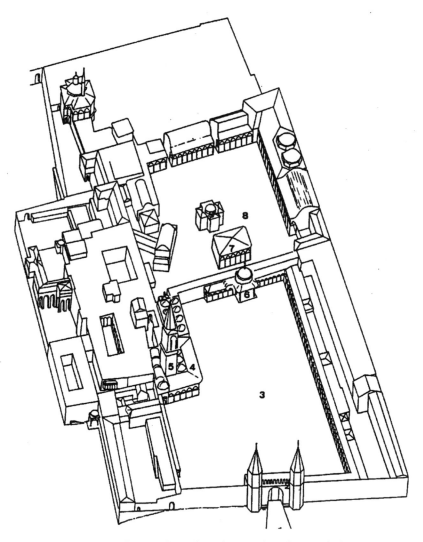

Figure 2. Drawing of Topkapı Palace in Istanbul

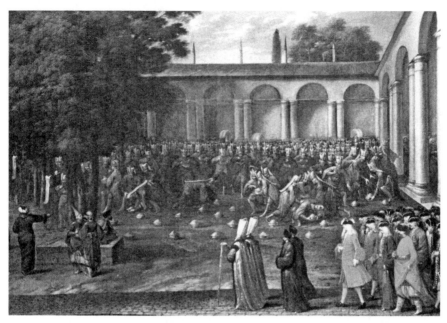

Figure 3. Painting of ambassador Cornelis Calkoen and his entourage
crossing the second courtyard of Topkapı Palace, by Jean-Baptiste Vanmour.
Amsterdam, Rijksmuseum A 4076

which are regarded as original works by Jean-Baptiste Vanmour. Seven
other 'Turkish' paintings probably did not belong to the bequest but came
from the headquarters of the Bureau of Levantine Trade in Amsterdam.[10]
In 2003 an exhibition which contained most of Vanmour's paintings from
the Calkoen Bequest was organized in the Rijksmuseum in Amsterdam and
was shown in 2004 in Topkapı Palace in Istanbul.[11]

Vanmour painted three pictures of Calkoen's audience at Topkapı
Palace. All three give interesting information about the ceremonial of am-
bassadorial visits to the Ottoman court. On the first painting (Rijksmuseum
A 4076, canvas 91.5 x 125 cm.) we can discern the Dutch ambassador and
his company crossing the enormous second court of the Topkapı Palace,
some 130 meters long and 110 meters wide, while some thousand soldiers
of the sultan's standing infantry, the Janissaries, threw themselves at bowls
of rice during *çanak yağması* (pot plundering) (Figure 2, no. 3, and Figure
3).[12] Diplomatic audiences with the sultan were traditionally held on the

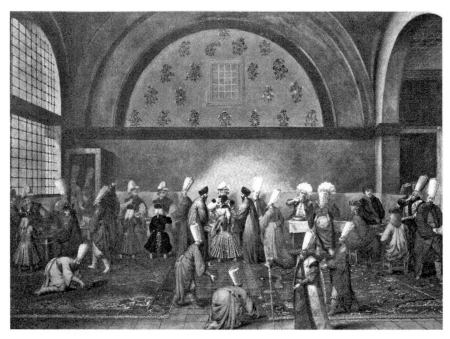

Figure 4. Painting of meal given by grand vizier in Topkapı Palace
in honour of ambassador Cornelis Calkoen, by Jean-Baptiste Vanmour.
Amsterdam, Rijksmuseum A 4077
(Detail of image below)

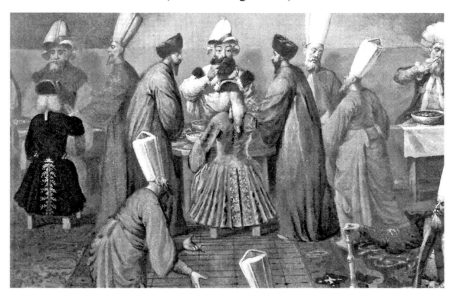

day that the Janissaries received their wages and dined at the palace. According to Calkoen's report, the Janissaries happily devoured a few loaves of bread and dishes with boiled rice (*pilav*), a scene which Calkoen interpreted as solemn proof of their loyalty and submission to the sultan. In short, the commotion made a deep impression on Calkoen, exactly as the sultan had intended.

Vanmour's second painting (Rijksmuseum A 4077, canvas 90 x 120 cm.) is even more revealing, because it depicts the lunch presented to Calkoen by the grand vizier in the name of Sultan Ahmed III (Figure 4). The Dutch ambassador was received by the grand vizier inside the Council Hall or Divan (Figure 2, no. 4), after which a meal was served from the imperial kitchens as a gesture of the sultan's hospitality towards his official guests.[13] Around three sides of the room there was a low couch covered with Turkish carpets (the divan from which the council took its name).

The *Relaes* gives a detailed description of the event. The meal was presented on low wooden stands which were covered with large round trays, made of silver, to serve as tables during the meal. On these trays pieces of bread and spoons, made of ivory or ebony, were put down for each diner. The food was served in large bowls, which were placed in the center of the tray. Everyone had to eat communally with his fingers from the same dish: *"dewelke soo schielijck worden opgenomen dat men ter nauwer nood de hand 2 of 3 mael daer in kan brengen"* (which was taken away so fast that one is only able to put one's hand in it no more than two or three times).[14] Calkoen was also astonished by the fact that his hosts did not use any plates or napkins. After the meal, which lasted for no more than half an hour, the diners washed their hands and drank coffee.[15] Furthermore, the Dutch guests received caftans not only as a token of the sultan's hospitality but also to cover the visitor's western clothing during their meeting with the sultan.

Finally, on Vanmour's third painting (Rijksmuseum A 4078, canvas 90 x 121 cm.) we can see Calkoen's actual audience with Sultan Ahmed III (Figure 5). The foreign envoy was taken through the Gate of Felicity (Figure 2, no. 6) into the Throne Room in the third court, where he was presented to the sultan (Figure 2, nos. 7 and 8). On a throne in the corner sat Sultan Ahmed III, with four princes at his side. Calkoen and his party were assisted by Ottoman courtiers. Calkoen's gifts were examined and the

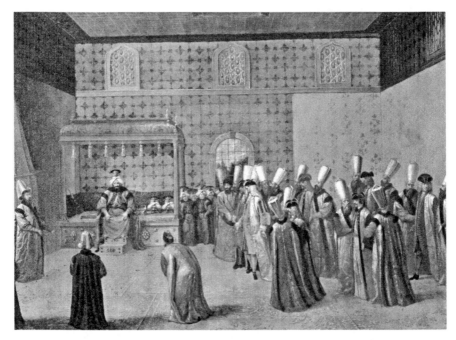

Figure 5. Painting of Ambassador Cornelis Calkoen in audience
with Sultan Ahmed III (1673-1736), by Jean-Baptiste Vanmour.
Amsterdam, Rijksmuseum A 4078

ambassador was introduced to the sultan.[16] (This offering of presents was
in fact part of a gift-counter gift ritual as the sultan also sent gifts to the
western Ambassadors. A decree issued by Sultan Mahmud I (r. 1730–54)
in 1749 mentions, for instance, the gift of 150 wild boars to the Dutch
Embassy in Istanbul.[17]) As a matter of fact, a first audience with the sultan
was the most important event for an ambassador in Istanbul and a kind of
initiation-ritual which involved a great show of strength of the sultan's
standing infantry, the Janissaries, and during which the envoy received a
mixture of humiliation and accolades.[18]

Apart from writing the *Relaes*, Cornelis Calkoen also left advice for
his successor at the Dutch Embassy, suggesting to him the types of food
which needed to be imported to Istanbul. According to Calkoen, the city
had all kinds and plenty of foodstuffs in many pleasant varieties. Nevertheless, he advised the new envoy to order every year from his home

country delicacies such as Dutch cheese, butter, smoked salmon, stockfish, salt cod, hams, sausages, grain, bread, powdered sugar, tea, potatoes, green peas, herring, rum, arrack, snuffing tobacco, and—last but not least— French wines or other fine wines of all varieties.[19] We know, for instance, from the seventeenth-century Dutch traveler Gerard Hinlopen that the Dutch resident's household consumed some 80 barrels of wine on a yearly basis, which according to Hinlopen showed that "the Dutch had the most splendid of all the European embassies in Istanbul."[20]

Dining Habits at the Ottoman Court

The formal banquets at the Ottoman court which were offered to ambassadors from Europe not only revealed the table customs in Topkapı Palace, but the degree of lavishness of the banquet was also a reflection of the relative status of the persons being honored.[21] The longer the meal lasted, the higher the visitor was regarded by the sultan. However, the meals were not only for the benefit of the foreign envoys. At the same time dishes with food were offered to the complete court entourage (including the Janissaries in the second court). This ostentatious public feeding was an important part of the court ceremonial, stressing the corporate unity of the palace household and its dependence on the sultan.

In the eighteenth century, when Cornelis Calkoen was received in audience by the sultan, the visitor was offered a meal immediately before his presentation to the sultan. However, three centuries earlier the order of ceremony was just the other way round. Initially, it was the Ottoman custom to offer a banquet to the foreign envoys directly after their official audience with the sultan.

The first description of such a dinner was written in 1433 by the French knight Bertrandon de la Brocquière (ca. 1400–1459) in his book *Le Voyage d'Outre-Mer*.[22] According to De la Brocquière, all the guests sat on the ground and ate from a round thin cloth, made of leather (a so-called *sofra*). On this were placed metal dishes filled with rice and meat. Curiously, the meal did not include bread or drink. The host, Sultan Murad II (r. 1421– 44, 1446–51), was the only person who got a long silk cloth, a napkin, and two big golden plates with meat. He was dining separately in the same room, but he was eating and drinking very little. It looked as if his presence at this dinner was more symbolic than to satisfy his appetite.[23]

Murad's successor to the throne, Sultan Mehmed II (r. 1444–46, 1451–81), however, no longer wished to eat together with his subjects. He preferred to dine only in the company of persons "of royal blood."[24] Since then, it was decided that all foreign ambassadors were presented with a meal by the grand vizier in the Council Hall (or Divan) before the official audience with the sultan.

Another revolutionary change in the dining protocol of the Ottoman court was the introduction of a circular tray (*sini*) on a wooden stand (Figure 6). This kind of table in an Occidental fashion was imposed by Sultan Suleyman the Magnificent (r. 1520–66) in the sixteenth century.[25] From this time on guests sat around these low circular trays and ate from communal dishes. The trays were not provided with plates, salt pots, knives, or forks. As a sixteenth-century German traveler rather bluntly remarked about the eating with fingers at the court, "Everything was just torn apart" (*alles wurde nur zerrissen*).[26] The only utensils used were serving ladles and soup spoons. Polish ambassadors and their retinues attending the Ottoman court were also completely preoccupied with the lack of knives and forks, describing the whole feast as a "scratching party."[27]

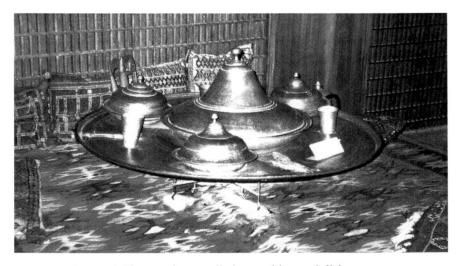

Figure 6. Picture of a so-called *sini* with metal dishes on top

Various embassy reports inform us that dishes were either set out together, regardless of ingredients, or served in quick succession.[28] This style of serving was followed at all social levels; the only difference between the elite and the common folk being the quantity and quality of textiles, utensils, and ingredients as well as of course the number of dishes.[29] The food was usually brought to the table in large bowls, copper dishes, covered pans or lidded porcelain dishes, which were placed in the center. Everyone ate with their spoons or fingers from the same dish.

If we are interested to know what kind of food people were eating with their fingers, it is good to consult registers listing the food served by the kitchens of Topkapı Palace, which have been published by Ottoman historians such as Ömer Lütfi Barkan, Günay Kut, Stéphane Yérasimos, Tülay Artan, and Hedda Reindl-Kiel.[30] Reindl-Kiel's study of some food records shows that ceremonial meals served in the seventeenth century mostly included chicken soup, chicken, and rice cooked in various ways.[31] Lamb was not yet the favored palace food and was reserved for special occasions. Apparently, this was the other way around two hundred years later, as Özge Samancı has shown in her work on nineteenth-century Ottoman upper-class cuisine.[32] Furthermore, freshly baked white bread, made of wheat, was also on the menu during the seventeenth century.[33] Fish and beef, though, were hardly served. For dessert, fruit, sweetmeats, and nuts were served on porcelain plates. During the banquet only persons of the highest rank drank *sherbet*, sweetened water flavored with rosewater or lemon; the rest had to slake their thirst with water. After the meal the diners washed their hands and drank coffee.

An additional banquet was served to lesser members of the ambassador's retinue who were not deemed worthy to eat in the Council Hall. Their food was served outside in one of the courtyards of the palace. According to the sixteenth-century diplomat and scholar Guillaume Postel (1510–1581), a long carpet was unrolled to accommodate the diners. The carpet was large enough to seat all those invited and offered enough space for a great number of porcelain dishes. A large crowd of soldiers, Janissaries, and other palace attendants assembled to gaze silently and motionlessly at the spectacle of the foreigners dining.[34]

There were many rules of etiquette relating to food and eating in Ottoman times, often derived from Islamic doctrine. These included washing the hands before and after meals, using three fingers to pass the food from dish to mouth, using two hands to break the bread, not smacking the lips, not looking at what one's neighbor was eating, turning one's head away from the table when coughing or sneezing, not talking with food in the mouth, etc.[35] Meal-times fitted in with the daily ritual of prayer and were of special importance within Islam, where the communal consumption of food is a recommended activity according to a *hadith*, which records that the Prophet remarked "Eat together with your family, since communal meals are blessed."[36]

Spoons were of foremost importance for eating soup or compote, and they came in many shapes and sizes. Often they were kept in carved or painted wooden spoon holders or embroidered bags known as *kaşıklık*. At the Ottoman court there was even a hierarchy in the use of spoons. A receipt from 1729 about the acquisition of spoons for the sultan shows that there were spoons for "normal" dishes such as soup and rice, as well as special spoons for compote, eggs, and rose jam.[37] These spoons for the elite were sometimes made from gold, silver, tortoiseshell, mother-of-pearl, or sandalwood (which was very expensive), and set with coral, ivory, or even precious stones.

Ottoman miniatures give some idea of how these spoons were used. At a banquet depicted in the *sûrnâme* of Sultan Ahmed III, individual spoons are placed in front of each guest, while there is a large serving tureen of soup at the center of the table (Figure 7). There was even an intricate etiquette of eating soup communally, whereby the right side of the spoon was only used to dish the broth up and the left side to eat from.[38]

Palace registers often list the quantities of porcelain plates, earthenware bowls, and metal dishes purchased for formal banquets at Topkapı Palace.[39] From one register we learn that each table was laid with twenty-seven serving dishes, six pans, and fourteen trays.[40] While some tables sat six or seven guests and others sat three or four people, there were also tables laid on the ground for one hundred people each. In all 80,000 plates, bowls, and dishes could be used.[41]

During public banquets for the ambassadors in the Divan there was an age-old tradition of carrying the food in silver and porcelain dishes from the imperial kitchens to the sultan's private residence and to the Council Hall. In 1599 the Austrian-Hungarian diplomat Baron Wenceslas Wratislaw

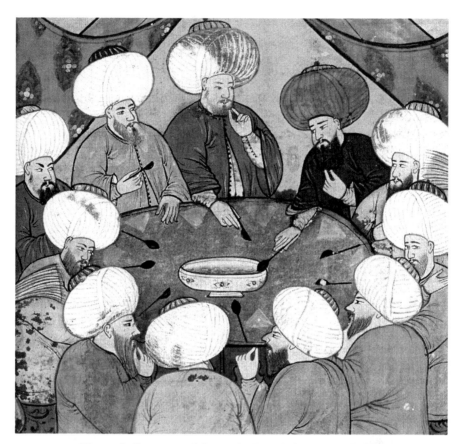

Figure 7. Ottoman miniature by Levnî, *Surnâme-i Vehbi*,
Topkapı Palace Museum Library (fol. 50a), 1712 AD

(1576–1635) described the ingenious way in which servants would file in
carrying the food from the kitchen:

> First came about 200 cup-bearers, or servers, . . . who placed them-
> selves in a row from the kitchen to the Sultan's apartment. . . .
> When it was dinner time, the superintendent of the kitchen brought
> from the cook a porcelain dish, and another covered dish, handed
> it to the waiter nearest him, he to a third, and so on till it came to
> the one who stood nearest to the Emperor's apartment. There,

again, stood other chamberlains, and one handed it to another, till the viands were carried very quickly, and without the slightest noise or clatter, to the Emperor's table.[42]

In addition, a similar row was formed to the table where the Council and foreign ambassadors were eating.

The Imperial Kitchens

The imperial kitchens, which extended along the right side of the second court at Topkapı Palace, formed a series of ten spacious chambers, each with a high dome and a conical chimney (Figure 8). The kitchen courtyard was separated from the second court by a steep wall above which rose the tall chimneys of the kitchens. At the north end of the narrow courtyard was the mosque of the royal kitchens, a small building with three domes. Adjacent to it were the confectionary kitchens (known as the Helvahâne), where fruit conserves, syrups, and sweets (such as *helva*) were made.

The ten kitchens, which had a staff of about 1500, all served different purposes. There were different kitchens for the sultan, followed by those for the queen mother (*valide* sultan), for the chief black eunuch and wives of the sultan, for the female officials and servants of the harem, and

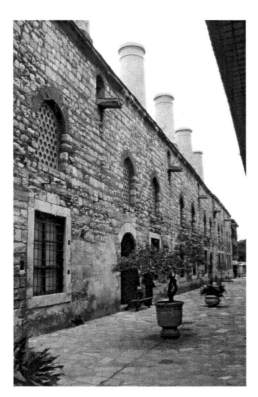

Figure 8. Imperial kitchens in Topkapı Palace

for the other classes of servants, officials, and guards.

Since the turn of the sixteenth century there were at least six hundred cooks at work in the imperial kitchens, assisted by a force of servants and "taste beforehands." They cooked with products in season, often with complicated cooking methods. There was a growing tendency to use luxurious foodstuffs. In 1527–28 the Ottoman court spent more than 2.3 million *akçe* on the imperial kitchens. In 1669–1670, 131 years later, the expenses of the imperial kitchens had risen to the remarkable sum of 52.5 million *akçe* (although inflation probably accounted for some of this increase, probably around 9.7 million *akçe* or 18 percent of the total sum).[43]

The kitchen complex also included a larder and a commissariat, where valuable ceramic tableware was stored. A number of documents contain references to the pottery store. Account books of 1527–29, for instance, mention the repair of this "ceramics room (*oda-ı çini*) near the imperial kitchens."[44] Here porcelains and celadon wares from China and the Far East were apparently stored together with the brightly colored local tin-glazed pottery from nearby Iznik. The porcelains and Iznik ceramic tableware used at the circumcision ceremonies of princes at the Hippodrome in 1582 were loaned out from the same storeroom.

However, the sultan's porcelains were better protected against earthquakes and fires than the less prestigious Iznik ceramics. Istanbul had many fires, which ravaged the city from the mid-fifteenth to the late nineteenth centuries.[45] This is one of the main reasons why so little Iznik pottery has survived to this day in Turkey. Furthermore, the sultan's passion for porcelains meant that it was costly, highly esteemed, and kept in well-protected cellars (so that there was very little in circulation). Thanks to this, Topkapı Palace now has the world's biggest collection of porcelains and celadon wares from China and the Far East after Peking and Dresden: ca. 10,700 pieces have survived to the present day and are now exhibited in the imperial kitchens complex (Figure 9).[46]

Unfortunately, not a trace of Iznik pottery remains in this collection. Iznik plates were evidently not good enough for the sultan, who preferred to eat off silver or gold plates, or green celadon wares, which were thought both to detect and neutralize poison.[47] As a result of this, the nicest and most complete pieces of Iznik ware can now be seen in western collections, for instance, in the Victoria & Albert Museum and the British Museum in London.

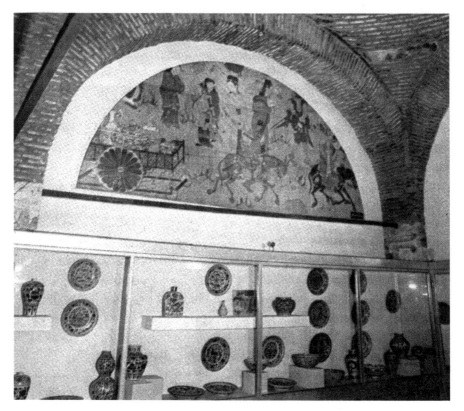

Figure 9. Porcelain collection in imperial kitchens in Topkapı Palace

Iznik Ware

The almost complete absence of Iznik pottery from Topkapı Palace today—
we have only broken pieces from excavations in contrast to the large quantities of Chinese porcelain surviving there—means that we have to rely
almost entirely on documentary references in order to establish whether—
and to what extent—Iznik pottery was used at the sultan's court in particular and in the rest of Ottoman Empire in general (Figure 10).[48]

Ottoman documents that have been examined up to now and shed light
on this question consist of schedules of fixed prices, probate inventories,
and various palace registers such as treasury accounts, stocktaking records,
sale registers, imperial kitchen records, and inventories of gifts. The earliest

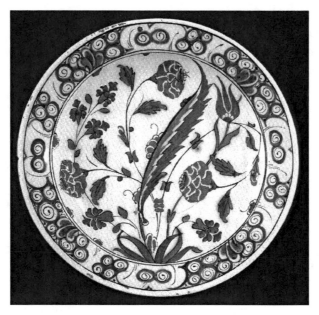

Figure 10. Plate of Iznik ware, Benaki Museum, Athens

document mentioning Iznik ceramics as being in use at Topkapı Palace can be dated to1489–90.[49] This register lists the types, quantities and prices of items, including Iznik pottery, purchased for the imperial kitchens. We learn from it that the cost of ninety-seven Iznik vessels was at that time 1,916 *akçe*.

Another kitchen record from 1582 provides evidence for special occasions. For example, during the festivities for the circumcision of the son of Sultan Murad III, which lasted fifty-two days and nights, 541 extra Iznik plates, dishes, and bowls were purchased from the bazaar to supplement the Chinese porcelain, copperware, and Iznik ceramics that were brought out of the imperial kitchens. According to Atasoy and Raby, this means that a great deal of Iznik pottery was available on the open market and that the Palace preferred to buy its Iznik vessels from the merchants in the Istanbul bazaar rather than from the potters themselves.[50]

Unlike foreign buyers, the Ottoman court paid fixed prices that were pegged to an artificially low scale for these wares. In an account from

1617–18 the prices of 6,331 types of Iznik ceramics range from 60.70 *akçe* for a large jar to only 2 *akçe* for a small cup. As a result, the Iznik potters increasingly preferred to make vessels for sale on the open market rather than ceramics on commission for the court. A royal decree sent to Iznik in 1585 ordered ceramic workshops to stop making tableware for the open market and turn their energies toward making tiles for Topkapı Palace in Istanbul.[51]

The documents also show that Iznik ware was mainly used as an everyday ware. Even in the sixteenth century, when the quality of the texture and decoration of Iznik ceramics reached its peak, the Ottoman sultans preferred the more expensive and valuable foreign wares (such as Chinese porcelains). The archival sources suggest that Iznik ware was stored in large quantities in the imperial kitchens of Topkapı Palace, ready for use on a day-to-day basis. The documents refer to "compote bowls," "large yoghurt bowls," "salad and sweetmeat dishes," "lamb dishes," and even to "dishes for various puddings," or "for clotted cream."[52]

Prices and quantities in the probate inventories of Edirne's wealthy residents seem to indicate that, compared with Chinese porcelain, Iznik pottery was cheap and widely available.[53] The potter's skill and the taste of the decoration made them an acceptable substitute for porcelain and for metal, too. There is ample evidence for the importance of Iznik pottery in fine houses as opposed to vessels of wood, base metal (brass or copper), porcelains, or even metal. It has rightly been suggested that at the Ottoman court Iznik ceramics and Chinese porcelain perhaps filled the gap between wood, tinned copper, or crude kitchen wares on the one hand, and gold and silver on the other.[54]

Kütahya Ware

In the seventeenth and eighteenth centuries, at the time whenn Cornelis Calkoen was living in Istanbul, the ceramic industry at Kütahya, about 200 km. southeast of Istanbul in northwestern Anatolia, occupied the leading position previously [or, that had been] held by Iznik (Figure 11). Pottery making and tile manufacture had started here around the same time as in Iznik. Entries for 1444–45 and 1485–86 in the endowment registers for the

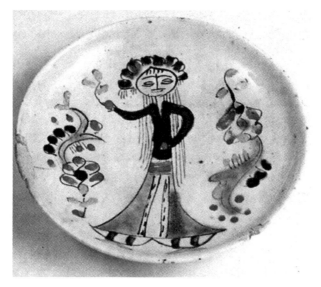

Figure 11. Plate of Kütahya ware, Çinili Kösk, Istanbul

Church of St. Mary in Kütahya give the names of two potters, showing that potteries existed there already in the fifteenth century.[55]

The ceramic workshops at Kütahya initially played a secondary role, providing Iznik with additional capacity when necessary. The fact that the Kütahya potteries were not very dependent on court patronage enabled them to remain economically viable. From an imperial edict written to the *kadı* (judge) of Kütahya in 1608 we learn that by this time there was even rivalry between the potters of Iznik and Kütahya. The *kadı* received instructions from Istanbul that the "cup-makers of Kütahya" should sell soda to the chief tile maker in Iznik at the price set by the government.[56]

Two government registers of fixed prices for the sale of various types of pottery have been published so far: one is dated September 15, 1600, the other December 31, 1640.[57] The pottery recorded in the 1600 schedule is arranged by type. Under the heading of "salad and sweetmeat dishes," the following prices of pottery from Iznik and Kütahya are given in the list of September 15, 1600 (see Table 1).

TABLE 1

New and old prices of Iznik and Kütahya wares in a 1600 list.

Salad and sweetmeat dishes	New price (in akçe)	Old price (in akçe)
Iznik ware	10	14
Kütahya ware	8 or 7	16

The list shows a puzzling (and as yet unexplained) reversal, the older Kütahya dishes being more expensive, and the newer ones (with the new regulated price) less expensive than the Iznik ones. It would be interesting to explore in the future whether this remarkable drop in prices could be related to new manufacture and decoration methods (perhaps related to mass-production), which resulted in a decline in quality of seventeenth century Kütahya ware.

Probate registers often list ceramics from Iznik and Kütahya together with Chinese porcelains in inventories of estates. They seem to show that Iznik pottery is always valued lower than Chinese porcelain, although in the inventory of the possessions of one Hacı Hürrem Bey, dated 1623, we find interestingly that a piece of Chinese porcelain is valued at 150 akçe, compared to 60 akçe for an Iznik dish and 500 akçe for a Kütahya dish.[58] There is, unfortunately, no additional information concerning this Kütahya dish, which might explain its remarkable high value by a possible exceptional size, date, or quality.

The most distinctive products of Kütahya were thinly-potted, polychrome painted vessels in a fine, whitish fritware. Small coffee cups (often with matching saucers), bowls, jugs, and coffee pots made up the majority of production (Figure 12). The shapes of the coffee cups were probably taken from Chinese porcelains or from porcelains made at Vienna and Meissen (Germany) about 1730–40.[59]

In the written sources of the time we see references to the use of this sort of coffee cup. In 1839 the Western traveller Ami Boué (1794–1881) described the serving of coffee in the Ottoman Empire, apparently refering to Kütahya ware: "*Der Kaffee wird in sehr kleinen, weissen Porzellantassen*

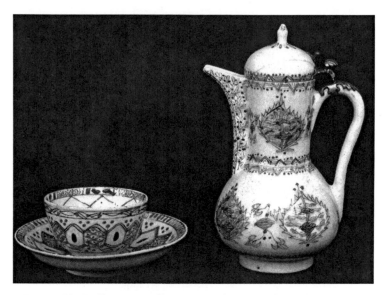

Figure 12. Coffee pot, coffee cup, and saucer of Kütahya ware,
Çinili Kösk, Istanbul

... aufgetragen, welche oftmals mit einem feinen Goldrand, aber nur bei sehr reichen Leuten mit Malereien verziert sind" (The coffee is served in very small cups made of porcelain ... which are often decorated with a fine golden rim, but only very rich people have them with painted decoration).[60]

The delicacy of the Kütahya cups suggests that they were also made for intimate gatherings in Ottoman society and not only for the robust public use in coffee houses and bazaars. Coffee drinking had become a sort of national pastime in the eighteenth century.[61] Coffee was not only drunk in coffeehouses but also in the harem, in the *hamam* (bathhouse), and at garden parties and picnics.

Remarks on the consumption of coffee are, for instance, frequent in Lady Mary Wortley Montagu's famous Turkish letters, written while she accompanied her husband on a trip in 1718. She reported that after the end of meals she often was offered coffee served in small cups of "the finest China with soucoups of silver gilt or gold." There were sets of metal coffee pots, porcelain cups in filigree holders, and small dishes for offering coffee and refreshments to the guests. It has therefore been suggested that in the

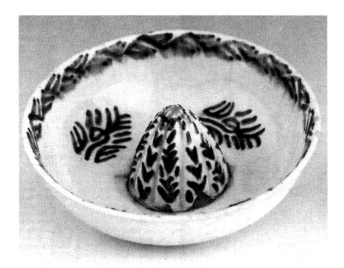

Figure 13. Lemon-squeezer of Kütahya ware,
Sadberk Hanim Museum, Istanbul

early eighteenth century Kütahya ware well suited the pleasure-seeking, romantic atmosphere that prevailed among the wealthy classes during the "Tulip Age" of the Ottoman Empire.[62]

Lemon-squeezers also were made at Kütahya in the first quarter of the eighteenth century (Figure 13).[63] Lemons were not grown in northern Anatolia, but we learn from various sources that lemons and lemon-juice were imported from the Aegean region to Istanbul in the seventeenth and eighteenth centuries for making lemon *sherbet*. This drink was a mixture of lemon juice, sugar, honey, and water, sometimes flavored with musk and ambergris, and often cooled with ice or snow. A simpler *sherbet* was made of water and with either honey or sugar.

The Distribution of Iznik and Kütahya Wares in the Provinces

The wares from Iznik and Kütahya were the direct result of improved pottery technology (compared to ceramics made in the fifteenth century), and they were apparently specifically designed for the tables of the upper and middle classes. Their glossy white surface, painted with metallic oxides, not only gave a colorful decoration but also proved easily adaptable to meet new design-trends in the most fashionable Renaissance and Islamic styles of the time.

Although tin-glazed pottery was a relatively expensive up-market product (tin had to be imported from abroad and was not cheap), these wares were always made primarily for daily use. In 1633 Evliya Çelebi (1611–ca. 1682) describes a parade of 300 merchants of pottery before Sultan Murad IV (r. 1623–40). According to the Ottoman traveller the merchants adorned their shops with "fayence of Nicaea (Iznik) and Kutahie."[64] Interesting in this respect are also Evliya Çelebi's remarks about the 20 "menders of broken cups," who paraded before the sultan while actually mending broken cups, and about the 25 craftsmen working in ten Istanbul workshops while clamping and pinning broken pots. This suggests that there was even an industry of recycling broken pottery (from Iznik and Kütahya?) during the seventeenth century.[65]

The colorful fine wares from Iznik and Kütahya were immensely popular, not only at home but also abroad, thanks to the thriving trade between the Ottoman Empire and the West. Fragments have been dug up in excavations from Fustat (old Cairo) in Egypt[66] to Waltham Abbey in Britain.[67] Iznik ware was sold by numerous retailers in Istanbul, where the Venetian and Genoese merchants had headquarters, and through Venice found its way into Germany and the north. We learn from the Journal of Stephan Gerlach (1546–1612), secretary and minister of the Austrian embassy to the Porte between 1573 and 1578, that his master David Ungnad had spent over one hundred ducats on pottery vessels and one thousand thalers on "Nicaean tiles" for shipment via Venice.[68]

Two other documents identify the trade of Kütahya vessels in the early eighteenth century. In one, from 1715, the French merchant and traveler Paul Lucas (1664–1737) lists, for instance, the types of Kütahya ware which he sent back to France from Istanbul: "*une douzaine des tasses à café avec leurs soucoupes, une tasse, deux bouteilles pour mettre de l'eau de rose, deux salières et deux escritoires, le tout de porcelaine de Cutajé.*"[69] Another Frenchman, Claude Charles de Peyssonnel (1727–1790), French Consul in the Crimea in 1753, lists among the products traded there each year, "*environs deux cents paniers de fayence de Cutahié de tout espèce, comme pots, vases de toutes grandeurs, tasses à sorbet et à café, etc.*"[70]

Excavations and field surveys in Greece have revealed that Iznik and Kütahya ceramics were also known in this part of the Ottoman Empire.[71] Although not abundant, pieces of pottery from Iznik and Kütahya have been found at Athens,[72] at Skyros,[73] at Thessaloniki,[74] at Kalapodi in Lokris,[75] and at two rural sites in Boeotia.[76] These wares have also been excavated at Nicosia and Kouklia on Cyprus.[77]

In addition, fragments of bowls and dishes from Iznik and Kütahya were found in some sixteenth–eighteenth century rubbish pits at an excavation in the historical center of Thebes.[78] The presence and quality of these

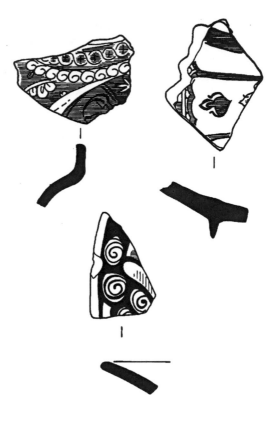

Figure 14. Fragments of Iznik ware, found at excavations in Greece

ceramics in the Theban waste pits appear to represent the discards of a well-to-do urban household which was able to import decorative tableware from the Ottoman Empire (Figures 14–15).

Apart from these excavated finds we also have the *bacini* as a source of information about the distribution of Iznik and Kütahya pottery. *Bacini* is the Italian term for decorated bowls which were embedded in church façades in both Italy and Greece from the eleventh century. In Greece, the custom remained popular into Ottoman times. *Bacini* of this period (including examples of Iznik and Kütahya pottery) were inlaid in the walls of several churches in Attica, near Chalkis on Evvia, on Mount Athos, and on

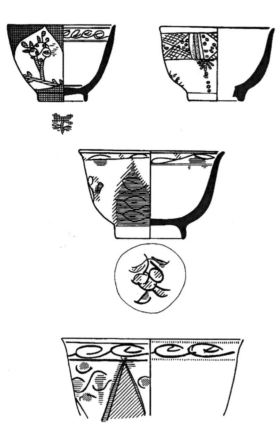

Figure 15. Fragments of Kütahya ware, found at excavations in Greece

the islands of Salamis and Hydra.[79]

All in all, it is clear that the imports of Iznik and Kütahya pottery in Greek lands were no small matter. These new fashionable tin-glazed wares from the Ottoman Empire, which played such a large part in the dining ritual at the court of the sultan, gave new impetus to all sorts of developments in local ceramics in the provinces, most notably perhaps the Greek imitations of Iznik ware.

Archaeologists often concentrate on those things which survive best in the ground and therefore occur most frequently in the archaeological record, such as ceramics in post-medieval rubbish.[80] However, pottery finds represent often only a fraction of the actual range of products consumed. There are two reasons for this. First, some types of material decay more easily than others in the ground. Second, some materials were collected in the past for recycling, particularly metal and glass. So, a typical archaeological assemblage will largely comprise finds that do not fall into those two categories and, in fact, highlights the disparity between that which archaeologists recover and that which was actually consumed in the past.

It is, therefore, also worthwhile to see what the written sources can tell us about the use of daily-life objects in Ottoman times, compared to the

actual archaeological artefacts that we found in the ground. An analysis by
Colette Establet and Jean-Paul Pascual of thirty inheritance inventories
found in the Damascus *kadı* registers (*sicil*) shows whatever was present
in an Ottoman household in Damascus in the late seventeenth and early
eighteenth centuries.[81]

When we compare in Table 2 the number of items used in the preparation and consumption of food with those of personal objects such as clothes,
underwear, furnishings, arms, jewelry, or books, we note in the percentages
the importance of food- and drink-related objects (made of metal, glass and
pottery) in thirty modest households (44.5 %) and in the richer household
of a sheikh (36.5%).

TABLE 2

The importance of food and drink-related objects
within Ottoman households in late seventeenth- and early
eighteenth-century Damascus.[82]

Owner(s)	Number of domestic objects owned	Number of items linked to food and drink	Percentages
30 households together	3090	1375	44.5
1 sheik	4275	1555	36.5

However, as Table 3 shows, the relatively large number of food-and-
drink-related objects does not mean that the value of pots, pans, and crockery made up a significant share of anyone's fortune. Quite to the contrary:
the food-and-drink-related items were relatively cheap. In addition, the
items found in the wealthy home of a sheikh do not significantly differ in
value from those owned by more modest Damascus households. Well-to-
do families did accumulate large collections of crockery, pots, and pans.
Most of the latter were made of copper, which if damaged could easily be
melted down and recast. It is perhaps hardly a monumental surprise that
the more expensive metal vessels were often owned by men, whereas
women owned items made of glass and of crockery, such as fragile and
largely decorative dishes and cups.

The wealthy and modest Damascus households used more or less the same food-and-drink items; however, the materials from which these objects were made do vary according to the economic level of the household. Apparently, the quality of the ceramics with respect to texture, form, and decoration also served as a mark of distinction: the scribes took, for instance, particular note of a number of pieces made of Chinese porcelain, but Iznik ware (well past its prime in the seventeenth century) appears only in a single instance.

TABLE 3.

The monetary values of food- and drink-related objects (in *gurush*) within Ottoman households in late seventeenth- and early eighteenth-century Damascus.[83]

Owner(s)	Values of domestic objects owned	Values of food-and drink-related items	Percentage (food-and drink-related items to total of domestic objects)	Average values of food-and drink-related items
30 households together	6688	1154	17.2	0.83
1 sheik	7730	1321	17.1	0.87

Conclusion

If we try to reconstruct Cornelis Calkoen's lunch in Topkapı Palace on Sunday, September 14, 1727, it is clear that his banquet was held at the Council Hall in the second court before his official audience with Sultan Ahmed III. The Dutch ambassador surely had to eat from a *sini*, sitting on a low couch covered with carpets (see Table 4).

According to Calkoen's report to his principals in Amsterdam, he had to eat from a communal dish with only three fingers. Obviously this happened with his right hand according to Islamic doctrine (although this was not mentioned specifically by Calkoen). The Islamic culinary laws also demanded that the diners did not use knives to cut their meat but broke and ate it with their fingers. Furthermore, all the guests were forced to eat in a hurry.

Freshly baked white bread was laid on the *sini* for each diner, but there were no individual plates or napkins. The only utensils used were spoons, often beautifully made of ivory or ebony, for eating soup and compote. Calkoen and his fellow-diners had to follow the intricate etiquette of eating soup communally, whereby the right side of these spoons was used only to dish the liquid up and the left side to eat from it.

The dishes were handed over by court servants, forming a row from the imperial kitchens (next to the Second Court) to the *sini* where Calkoen was eating. His lunch was probably prepared by many professional cooks in the kitchens of the sultan.

On the menu were probably rice and chicken, and the food was served in large dishes made of silver and China porcelain. Perhaps the diners also ate from cheaper, everyday ware made at Iznik, although the heyday of this pottery center was already over by the eighteenthth century.

After the lunch, the diners washed their hands and drank coffee. Perhaps the coffee was served in decorative coffee cups, made at Kütahya, which were very popular among the Ottoman elite in the eighteenth century. In addition, the lemon *sherbet*, the only drink offered during the meal, could have been made in the imperial kitchens from lemons pressed with lemon squeezers—these last made at Kütahya, of course.

Both Iznik ware and Kütahya ware were the result of improved pottery technology and apparently specifically designed for the table of the Ottoman upper classes. It is, therefore, no coincidence that Cornelis Calkoen probably ate from an Iznik dish and certainly drank his coffee from a Kütahya cup.

Taking into account all well-known methodological *caveats*, traveler's accounts may provide us with unique insights into matters of daily life of visited countries. It seems that Ambassador Cornelis Calkoen's apparently accurate description of his audience with the sultan not only reveals a typical reaction of westerners to Ottoman palace cuisine, but also gives a valuable insight in what actually did strike him as 'peculiar' (that is: 'un-European') in the Ottoman dining culture. Calkoen notes specifically as "different" that his hosts were eating quickly and communally from large bowls placed in the center of a tray, as well as that they were eating with their fingers without the use of napkins, forks, or knives. This last characteristic was also observed by other foreign envoys, who sometimes outright condemned this feature of Ottoman eating habits.

It is significant that western guests at the Ottoman court apparently considered dining manners as markers of distinction between the West and the Orient, rather than the lavish choice and quantity of the dishes, the ingredients, or the dining equipment (these last items being matters of prestige for the Ottoman court). In this respect, the same festive meals are viewed in a distinctly different perspective in the European documents compared to the Ottoman ones, and consequently they offer a valuable side window to look at Ottoman social history.

TABLE 4

Calkoen's lunch in Topkapı Palace on
Sunday, September 14, 1727: The main characteristics.

- Eating from a low round table (*sini*) and sitting on a low stool
- Eating with the fingers from a communal dish
- No knives or forks, using only spoons for liquid dishes
- No individual plates or napkins
- Rice and chicken served in large communal dishes made of porcelain or silver
- Drinking *sherbet* during the meal and coffee after dinner

Notes

1. J. Goody, *Cooking, Cuisine and Class. A Study in Comparative Sociology* (Cambridge: Cambridge University Press, 1982), p. 128; S. Mennel, *All Manners of Food: Eating and Taste in England and France from the Middle Ages to the Present* (Oxford: Basil Blackwell, 1985). All the dates in the text refer to the period after Christ and are given in the Gregorian calendar.

2. See for a similar phenomenon concerning ancient Persian cuisine, H. Sancisi-Weerdenburg, "De oorsprong van een 'haute cuisine," *Phoenix* 43, no. 2 (1997): pp. 93–102.

3. The full title of Calkoen's description of his audience to the Ottoman court is "Relaes van het gepasseerde in de publique audiëntien van zijne excellentie mijnheere Cornelis Calkoen, ambassadeur van weegens haer Hoog Mogende

de Heeren Staaten Generael der Verenigde Neederlanden bij zijn Sultannise Majestijt Achmet Ghan de derde van die naem" (Report of all things which happened during the public audience of his excellency Mister Cornelis Calkoen, ambassador of the splendid lords of the States General of the Dutch Republic at his Sultanic Majesty Ahmed Khan III of that name). This document can be found in the Algemeen Rijksarchief (The Hague) or ARA, Familiearchief Calkoen, 561.

4. According to G. R. Bosscha Erdbrink, *At the Threshold of Felicity: Ottoman-Dutch Relations During the Embassy of Cornelis Cakoen at the Sublime Porte 1726–1744* (Ankara: Türk Tarih Kurumu Basimevi, 1975), p. 77, the first member of his family adopted around 1600 the name 'Calkoen' (*lit.* turkey) because of the sign hanging over his cloth shop with the title "*In den blaeuwen Calkoen*" (*lit.* In the Blue Turkey). Apart from cloth the family's commercial interest was also in Mediterranean trade and dyeing.

5. Bosscha Erdbrink, *At the Threshold of Felicity*, p. 81; A. Abelmann, "Cornelis Calkoen op audiëntie bij sultan Ahmed III," in *Topkapi en turkomanie: Turks-Nederlandse ontmoetingen sinds 1600*, ed. H. Theunissen, A. Abelmann and W. Meulenkamp (Amsterdam: Bataafsche Leeuw, 1989), p. 27; see also R. E. O. Ekkart and Q. Buvelot, *Hollanders in beeld – Portretten in de Gouden Eeuw* (The Hague: Mauritshuis, 2007), pp. 200–203 for Rembrandt's painting of Jan Six (Amsterdam, Collection Six).

6. E. Sint Nicolaas, "The Ambassador and the Sultan", in *The Ambassador, the Sultan and the Artist. An Audience in Istanbul* (Amsterdam and Zwolle: Rijksmuseum & Waanders, 2003), p. 15, fig. 14; M. Hoenkamp-Mazgon, *Palais de Hollande in Istanbul: The Embassy and Envoys of The Netherlands since 1612* (Amsterdam and Istanbul: Boom, 2002).

7. Nowadays, Beyaz Gül is immortalised in stone in the garden of the present Dutch Consulate, and according to some of its inhabitants, her ghost regularly wanders through the building of the Dutch Consulate at night.

8. See J. Slot, "De diplomatieke betrekkingen tussen Nederland en het Osmaanse Rijk", in *Topkapı en turkomanie; Turks-Nederlandse ontmoetingen sinds 1600*, ed. H. Theunissen, A. Abelmann and W. Meulenkamp (Amsterdam: Bataafsche Leeuw, 1989), p. 14.

9. R. van Luttervelt, *De 'Turkse' schilderijen van J.B. Vanmour en zijn school: De verzameling van Cornelis Calkoen, ambassadeur bij de Hoge Porte, 1725-1743* (Istanbul: Nederlands Historisch Archeologisch Instituut in het Nabije Oosten, 1958); G. Irepoğlu, *Levni: Painting, Poetry, Colour* (Istanbul: Republic of Turkey Ministry of Culture, 1999), pp. 26-29; E. Sint Nicolaas, D. Bull, G. Renda and G. Irepoğlu, *An Eyewitness of the Tulip Era: Jean-Baptiste Vanmour* (Istanbul: Koçbank, 2003). Most paintings of Jean-Baptiste Vanmour

were shown at an exhibition held in 2003 at the Rijksmuseum in Amsterdam and in 2004 at Topkapi Palace in Istanbul. See *The Ambassador, the Sultan and the Artist. An Audience in Istanbul* (Amsterdam/Zwolle: Rijksmuseum & Waanders, 2003) for the catalogue of this exhibition.

10. See P. J. J. van Thiel, *Alle schilderijen van het Rijksmuseum te Amsterdam: Volledig geïllustreerde catalogus* (Amsterdam and Haarlem: Rijksmuseum, 1976), p. 741 with more information on the history of this collection.

11. See *The Ambassador* and Sint Nicolaas *et al., An Eyewitness of the Tulip Era.*

12. Apparently, Cornelis Calkoen was accompanied by his secretary Jean-Luis Rigo, his dragoman Carlo Karatza, and a group of merchants and persons under Dutch protection; cf. Sint Nicolaas, "The ambassador and the Sultan," p. 6. A similar scene of 'pot plundering' was also described by the Dutch traveler, Johan Raye, heer van Breukelerwaart (1737–1823) during his audience with Sultan Mustafa III (1717–74) in *Een levenslustig heer op reis naar de Oriënt. Brieven van Johan Raye, heer van Breukelerwaart 1764-1769* (Baarn: Bosch and Keuning, 1987), p. 55. According to Raye, the Janissaries were trampled in their haste to get to the bowls of *pilav* (rice with mutton and spices) with the effect of spilling most dishes and covering the faces of the soldiers with rice.

13. Cf. K. Dilger, *Untersuchungen zur Geschichte des Osmanischen Hoffzeremoniells im 15. und 16. Jahrhundert* (Munich: Rudolph Trofenik, 1967), pp. 104–21 and G. Necipoğlu, *Architecture, Ceremonial, And Power: The Topkapı Palace in the Fifteenth and Sixteenth Centuries* (Cambridge, MA, and London: The Architectural History Foundation, 1991), pp. 55 and 72 for this old tradition of the Ottoman dynasty.

14. ARA, Familiearchief Calkoen, 561.

15. Not all foreign envoys enjoyed the drinking of coffee, as is shown in S. Westerberg, "Claes Rålamb: Statesman, Scholar and Ambassador," in *The Sultan's Procession: The Swedish Embassy to Sultan Mehmed IV in 1657–1658 and the Rålamb Paintings*, ed. K. Ådahl (Istanbul: Pera Museum, 2006), p. 39, and C. Kafadar, "The City That Rålamb Visited: The Political and Cultural Climate of Istanbul in the 1650s," in *The Sultan's Procession: The Swedish Embassy to Sultan Mehmed IV in 1657–1658 and the Rålamb Paintings*, ed. K. Ådahl (Istanbul: Pera Museum, 2006), p. 69 and note 25 with respect to the seventeenth-century Swedish ambassador Claes Rålamb.

16. Calkoen's gifts included, amongst others, high-quality waistcoats made of Dutch woolen cloth, satin, and velvet; a crystal cabinet; two silver filigree flowerpots with flowers made of cloth; a small cabinet containing costly scented oils; a pair of binoculars; four pairs of spectacles in an exquisite case and twelve porcelain pots filled with various candied spices; see also Sint Nicolaas, "The Ambassador and the Sultan," pp. 10-11, fig. 8.

17. ARA, Legatiearchief Turkije 1668-1811.1090; cf. A. H. De Groot, *The Nether-lands and Turkey: Four Hundred Years of Political, Economical, Social and Cultural Relations. Selected Essays* (Istanbul: Artpress, 2007), p. 44 for a pic-ture of this decree. See also A. H. De Groot, *The Ottoman Empire and the Dutch Republic: A History of the Earliest Diplomatic Relations 1610–1630* (Leiden: Nederlands Instituut voor het Nabije Oosten, 1978), and M. Bulut, *Ottoman-Dutch Economic Relations in the Early Modern Period 1571–1699* (Ph.D. diss., University of Utrecht, 2000), for earlier diplomatic and economic Ottoman-Dutch relations.

18. Slot, "De diplomatieke betrekkingen," p. 11; see also in general, Dilger, *Un-tersuchungen zur Geschichte.*

19. ARA, 2de afd. Familiearchief Van Dedem van Gelder, aanwinsten 1913–1917. See also Abelmann, "Cornelis Calkopen op audiëntie," p. 35 and note 42.

20. J. Oddens pers. comm.

21. It was customary among envoys to document these audiences, both in a writ-ten account and with painted images (often executed in a formalized manner). See also M. Laine, "Audienstavlorna på Biby," in *Minnet av Konstantinopel: Den osmansk-turkiska 1700-tallssamlingen på Biby*, ed. K. Ådahl *et al.* (Stockholm: Atlantis, 2003), pp. 113–45, and K. Ådahl, "Claes Brorson Rålamb's Embassy to the Sublime Porte in 1657–1658," in *The Sultan's Pro-cession: The Swedish Embassy to Sultan Mehmed IV in 1657–1658 and the Rålamb Paintings*, ed. K. Ådahl (Istanbul: Pera Museum, 2006), pp. 8-25 for written documents of audiences of the Swedish envoys Gustaf and Ulric Cels-ing and Claes Rålamb illustrated with commemorative paintings and plans of the Topkapı Palace.

22. Dilger, *Untersuchungen zur Geschichte*, p. 105.

23. Dilger, *Untersuchungen zur Geschichte*, p. 105.

24. Dilger, *Untersuchungen zur Geschichte*, p. 117.

25. Dilger, *Untersuchungen zur Geschichte*, p. 121.

26. S. Gerlach, *Stephan Gerlachs dess Aeltern Tage-buch der von zween ghar-würdigsten Römischen Käysern Maximiliano und Rudolpho Beyderseits den Andern dieses Nahmens, Höchstseeligster Gedächtnuss, an die Ottomanische Pforte zu Constantinopel Abgefertigten, und durch den Wohlgebohrnen Herrn Hn. David Ungnad, Freyherrn zu Sonnegk und Preyburg u. Römisch Kayser-liche Raht Mit Würcklicher Erhalt und Verlangerung dess Friedens zwischen den Ottomanischen und Römischen Kayserthum und demselben angehörigen Landen und Köningreichen u. Glücklichst vollbrachter Gesandschaft auf denen Gerlachischen Zeit Seiner hierbey bedienten Hoff-Prediger-Ampts-Stelle, eygenhandig auffgesetzten und nachgelassenen Schriften, herfür gege-*

ben durch Seinen Enckel M. Samuelem Gerlachium Special-Superintendenten zu Gröningen in dem hertzogthum Würtenberg. Mit eine Vorrede Herrn Tobiae Wagneri der H. Schrift D. und Prof. auch Cantzlers bey der Hohen-Schul, und Propstes der Kirchen zu Tübingen (Frankfurt am Main: Johann-David Zunners, 1674), p. 283.

27. D. Kolodziejczyk, "Polish Embassies in Istanbul, or: How to Sponge on Your Host Without Losing Your Self-esteem," in *The Illuminated Table, The Prosperous House*, ed. S. Faroqhi and C.K. Neumann, (Würzburg: Ergon Verlag, 2003), p. 55. Apparently, also the Swedish ambassador had the same experience; cf. Laine, "Audienstavlorna på Biby."

28. See H. Reindl-Kiel, "Die Lippen der Geliebten: Betrachtungen zur Geschichte der türkischen Küche," *Mitteilungen der Deutsch-Türkische Gesellschaft* 116 (2003): p. 61 and note 9, mentioning the seventeenth-century diplomat Paul Rycaut who referred to dishes at a banquet being quickly served one and another "taken off to make room for another."

29. J. Scarce, *Domestic Culture in the Middle East: An Exploration of the Household Interior* (Edinburgh: National Museums of Scotland, 1996). The eighteenth-century Dutch traveler John Raye in *Een levenslustig heer*, pp. 55 and 57, mentioned at least thirty-four dishes of food served during his audience with Sultan Mustafa III (1717–74). However, he regarded the food, consisting of merely bread, rice, roasted meat en sweets, as "not very luxurious."

30. See S. Faroqhi, "Introduction," in *The Illuminated Table, The Prosperous House* ed. S. Faroqhi and C.K. Neumann (Würzburg: Ergon Verlag, 2003), pp. 9–33, with further literature.

31. Reindl-Kiel, "Die Lippen der Geliebten."

32. Ö. Samancı, "Culinary Consumption Patterns of the Ottoman Elite During the First Half of the Nineteenth Century," in *The Illuminated Table, The Prosperous House*, ed. S. Faroqhi and C.K. Neumann (Würzburg: Ergon Verlag, 2003), 161–84; Ö. Samancı, "19. Yüzyıl Istanbul Mutfağı'nda Yeni Lezzeter," *Yemek ve Kültür* 6 (2006): pp. 86–96.

33. Reindl-Kiel, "Die Lippen der Geliebten," suggests that the sultan meant to offer his diners a foretaste of paradise in the shape of highly valued foods, and in doing so enhancing Topkapı Palace's image "as a spiritual center providing food to its devotees."

34. M. And, *Istanbul in the 16th Century: The City, The Palace, Daily Life* (Istanbul: Akbank, 1994), p. 143.

35. See H. Kindermann, ed., *Uber die guten Sitten beim Essen und Trinken: Das ist das Buch von Al-Ghazzali's Hauptwerk* (Leyden: Brill, 1964), for more examples.

36. As cited by N. Araz, "Eat sweet, talk sweet," in *Timeless Tastes: Turkish Culinary Culture*, ed. S. Arsel (Istanbul: Divan, 1996), p. 21.

37. Reindl-Kiel, "Die Lippen der Geliebten," pp. 21–22.

38. M. Ursinus, "Die Ess- und Trinkgewohnheiten der Osmanen," in *Türkische Kunst und Kultur aus osmanischer Zeit* (Recklinghausen: Museum für Kunsthandwerk der Stadt Frankfurt, 1985), pp. 155-58.

39. N. Atasoy and J. Raby, *Iznik: The Pottery of Ottoman Turkey* (London: Alexandria Press, 1989), pp. 30–32.

40. G. Kut, "Turkish culinary culture," in *Timeless Tastes: Turkish Culinary Culture*, ed. S. Arsel (Istanbul: Divan, 1996), p. 48.

41. Kut, "Turkish Culinary Culture," p. 49.

42. As cited by Necipoğlu, *Architecture, Ceremonial, and Power*, p. 72.

43. Reindl-Kiel, "Die Lippen der Geliebten," p. 16.

44. Necipoğlu, *Architecture, Ceremonial and Power*, p. 72.

45. See Atasoy and Raby, *Iznik*, figs 1–2.

46. J. Vroom, *Byzantine to Modern Pottery in the Aegean: An Introduction and Field Guide* (Utrecht: Parnassus Press, 2005), p. 163. Apart from porcelains from China (ranging from the late Song Dynasty (13th c.). to the Qing Dynasty (1644–1912), the collection also includes celadon wares from China, porcelains from Japan and Turkey as well as imitation porcelains from Vietnam, Thailand, and Persia; cf. R. Krahl, N. Erbahar and J. Ayers, *Chinese Ceramics in the Topkapı Saray Museum, Istanbul: A Complete Catalogue* (New York: Sotheby's Publications, 1986), and T. Misugi, *Chinese Porcelain Collections in the Near East: Topkapı and Ardebil, Volume I* (Hong Kong: Hong Kong University Press, 1981).

47. M. Rogers, "Plate and its Substitutes in Ottoman Inventories," in *Pots & Pans: A Colloquium on Precious Metals and Ceramics in the Muslim, Chinese and Graeco-Roman Worlds*, ed. M. Vickers (Oxford: Oxford University Press, 1986), p. 117.

48. L. Caroll, "Toward an Archaeology of Non-elite Consumption in Late Ottoman Anatolia," in *A Historical Archaeology of the Ottoman Empire: Breaking New Ground*, ed. U. Baram and L. Caroll (New York: Kluwer Academic/Plenum Publishers, 2000), pp. 170–75; Vroom, *Byzantine to Modern Pottery*, 158–61.

49. Atasoy and Raby, *Iznik*, p. 30.

50. Atasoy and Raby, *Iznik*, p. 30.

51. See J. Vroom, *After Antiquity: Ceramics and Society in the Aegean from circa the 7th to the 20th centuries A.C. A Case Study from Boeotia, Central Greece*,

Archaeological Studies Leiden University 10 (Leiden: Leiden University, 2003), p. 296.

52. Atasoy and Raby, *Iznik*, pp. 43–47.

53. Atasoy and Raby, *Iznik*, pp. 25–27.

54. M. Rogers, "Archaeology vs. Archives: Some Recent Approaches to the Ottoman Pottery of Iznik," in *The Balance of Truth: Essays in Honour of Professor Geoffrey Lewis*, ed. Ç. Balım-Harding and C. Imber (Istanbul: Isis Press, 2000), pp. 275–92.

55. S. Akalin, "Kütahya Tiles and Pottery in a Historical Perspective," in *Delights of Kütahya* (Istanbul: Suna & Inan Kiraç, 1997), p. 10.

56. A. Lane, *Later Islamic Pottery: Persia, Syria, Egypt, Turkey*, 2nd ed. (London: Faber & Faber, 1971), p. 63; Akalin, "Kütahya Tiles and Pottery," p. 13.

57. Atasoy and Raby, *Iznik*, pp. 24–25; see also A.J. Carswell, "Kütahya Tiles and Ceramics," in *Turkish Tiles and Ceramics* (Istanbul: Sadberk Hanim Museum, 1991), p. 52; Akalin, "Kütahya Tiles and Pottery," p. 13.

58. Carswell, "Kütahya Tiles and Ceramics," p. 53; Akalin, "Kütahya Tiles and Pottery," p. 13.

59. A. Lane, "Turkish Peasant Pottery from Chanak and Kutahia," *The Connoisseur* 104 (1939): p. 236.

60. As cited by M. Ursinus, "Die Ess- und Trinkgewohnheiten der Osmanen," in *Türkische Kunst und Kultur aus osmanischer Zeit* (Recklinghausen: Museum für Kunsthandwerk der Stadt Frankfurt, 1985), p. 157.

61. J. Vroom, "Coffee and Archaeology: A Note on a Kütahya Ware Find in Boeotia, Greece," *Pharos (Journal of the Netherlands Institute at Athens)* 4 (1996): pp. 5–19; E. Işın, "Coffeehouses as Places of Conversation," in *The Illuminated Table, The Prosperous House,* ed. S. Faroqhi and C.K. Neumann (Würzburg: Ergon Verlag, 2003), pp. 199–208.

62. O. Watson, "Ceramics," in *Islamic Art in the Keir Collection*, ed. B.W. Robinson. (London: Faber Ltd), pp. 137–286; see also C. Finkel, *Osman's Dream: The Story of the Ottoman Empire 1300–1923* (London: John Murray, 2005), pp. 346–47 on the "Tulip Age."

63. A. J. Carswell, "The Lemon-Squeezer. A Unique Form of Turkish Pottery," in *IVème Congrès International d'Art Turc, 1971* (Aix-en-Provence: Éditions de l'Université de Provence 1976), pp. 29–45; Carswell, "Kütahya Tiles and Ceramics," p. 101, K. 132 from the Sadberk Hanim Museum in Istanbul.

64. Carswell, "The Lemon-Squeezer," p. 42; Carswell, "Kütahya Tiles and Ceramics," p. 53.

65. See Atasoy and Raby, *Iznik*, p. 37 and note 4; Vroom, *After Antiquity*, p. 283.

66. M. Azarnoush-Maillard, *Islamitisch aardewerk* (Brussel: Koninklijke Musea voor Kunst en Geschiedenis, 1977), p. 127, fig. 35c.

67. P. J. Huggins, "Excavations at Sewardstone Street, Walthan Abbey, Essex 1966," *Post-Medieval Archaeology* 3 (1969): p. 93, pl. 1; see also J. W. Hayes, *Excavations at Saraçhane in Istanbul, vol. II: The Pottery* (Washington, D.C.: Dumbarton Oaks, 1992), pp. 244–47 with further literature on the distribution of these wares.

68. Lane, *Later Islamic Pottery*, p. 58.

69. As cited by Lane, *Later Islamic Pottery*, p. 63.

70. As cited by Carswell, "Kütahya Tiles and Ceramics," p. 54.

71. Iznik and Kütahya pottery finds have also been excavated in the Crimea, Rumania, Bulgaria, Hungary, in the Adriatic (e.g., Dubrovnik and Muro Leccese in southern Italy) as well as on Cyprus. On Iznik and Kütahya finds outside Greece, see, for instance, Gh. I. Cantacuzino and Al. Radulescu, "Betrachtungen über die während dem Jahre 1971 im Kloster Putna geborgene Keramik," *Studii si cercetari de istorie veche* 25 (1974): pp. 527–44 (in Roumanian) for the Monastery of Putna in Roumania; G. Gerö, "Türkische Keramik in Ungarn, einheimische und importierten Waren," in *Fifth International Congress of Turkish Art*, ed. G. Feher (Budapest: Akademiai Kiado, 1978), pp. 363–84 for Budapest in Hungary (Gerö 1978); A. Margos, "Die Armenische Kirche Heiliger Stephanos in der Stadt Provadya," *Bulletin du Musée National de Varna* 12 (1976): pp. 137–39 (in Bulgarian) for Provadya in Bulgaria.

72. F. O. Waagé, "The Roman and Byzantine Pottery," *Hesperia* 2 (1933): pp. 279–328; M. A. Frantz, "Turkish Pottery from the Agora," *Hesperia* 11 (1942): pp. 1–28.

73. E. Pitari-Mayioletti, "Some European-made Treasures of Skyros," *Zygos* 4 (1973): pp. 6–9 (in Modern Greek).

74. E. Kourkoutidou, Chr. Tsioumi and Th. Pazaras, "Excavations at Thessaloniki," *Archaiologikon Deltion* 31 (1976 = 1984): pp. 267–70, pls. 210–13 (in Modern Greek); A. Vavylopoulou-Charitonidou, "Céramique d'offrande trouvée dans des tombes byzantines tardives de l'hippodrome de Thessalonique," in *Recherches sur la céramique byzantine* (*Bulletin du Correspondance Hellénique Suppl.* 18), ed. V. Déroche and J.-M. Spieser (Athens: École Française d'Athènes, 1989), pp. 209–25.

75. P. Armstrong, "The Byzantine and Later Pottery," in *Kalapodi: Ergebnisse der Ausgrabungen im Heiligtum der Artemis und des Apollon von Hyampolis in der antiken Phokis*, ed. R. C. S. Felsch (Mainz: Philipp von Zabern, 1996), pp. 336–71.

76. See Vroom, "Coffee and Archaeology;" J. Vroom, "Medieval and Post-Medieval Pottery from a Site in Boeotia: A Case Study Example of Post-Classical

Archaeology in Greece," *Annual of the British School at Athens* 93 (1998): pp. 513–46; J. Vroom, "Byzantine Garlic and Turkish Delight: Dining Habits and Cultural Change in Central Greece from Byzantine to Ottoman Times," *Archaeological Dialogues* 7 (2000): pp. 209–11; Vroom, *After Antiquity*, pp. 175–76 and 178; J. Vroom, "Breaking Pots: Medieval and Post-Medieval Ceramics from Central Greece," in *Medieval and Post-Medieval Greece: The Corfu Papers*, ed. J. Bintliff and H. Stöger (Oxford: Oxbow Books, 2009), p. 173.

77. A. H. S. Megaw, "Three Medieval Pit-Groups from Nicosia," *Report of Antiquities, Cyprus 1937-39* (1937 = 1951), pp. 145–68 and 224–26; M.-L. von Wartburg, "Types of Imported Table Ware at Kouklia in the Ottoman Period," *Report of the Department of Antiquities, Cyprus* (2001), pp. 366–67 and fig. 4.

78. J. Vroom, "Byzantine Garbage and Ottoman Waste," in E. Andrikou, V.L. Aravantinos, L. Godard, A. Sacconi, and J. Vroom, *Thèbes. Fouilles de la Cadmée II.2. Les tablettes en linéaire B de la 'Odos Pelopidou'. La céramique de la Odos Pelopidou et la chronologie du Linéaire B* 181-233 (Pisa and Rome: Institituti editoriali e poligrafici internazionali, 2006), pp. 181–233; J. Vroom, "Kütahya Between the Lines: Post-Medieval Ceramics as Historical Information," in *Between Venice and Istanbul: Colonial Landscapes in Early Modern Greece (Hesperia Supplement 40)*, ed. S. Davies and J. Davis (Princeton: The American School of Classical Studies at Athens, 2007), pp. 81–83, figs. 4.12–14.

79. E.g. A. J. Carswell, "Pottery and Tiles on Mount Athos," *Ars Orientalis* 6 (1966): pp. 77–90; G. A. Nikolakopoulos, "The Ceramics of the Chapel of Phaneromeni of Salamis," *Archaiologia* 28 (1988): 81–84 (in Modern Greek); G.A. Nikolakopoulos, "Embedded Ceramics of Churches," *Archaiologia* 33 (1989): pp. 66–71 (in Modern Greek); M. Kiel, "Byzantine Architecture and Painting in Central Greece 1460–1570," *Byzantinische Forschungen* 16 (1990): pp. 429-46; K. Korre-Zographou, *Ta kerameika tou Ellinikou chorou* (Athens: Ekdotikos Oikos Melissa, 1995), pp. 69–76 (in Modern Greek); see also Vroom, *After Antiquity*, p. 45.

80. D. H. Brown, "Class and Rubbish," in *Historical Archaeology: Back from the Edge*, ed. P. P. A. Funari, M. Hall and S. Jones (London and New York: Routledge, 1999), pp. 152–53.

81. C. Establet and J.-P. Pascual, "Cups, Plates, and Kitchenware in Late Seventeenth- and Early Eighteenth-Century Damascus," in *The Illuminated Table, The Prosperous Houseled.* S. Faroqhi and C.K. Neumann (Würzburg: Ergon Verlag, 2003), pp. 185–97.

82. Based on Establet and Pascual, "Cups, plates and kitchenware," table 2.

83. Based on Establet and Pascual, "Cups, plates and kitchenware," table 3.

Bibliography

Abd al-Karim b. Shaykh Musa. *Maqalat-i Sayyid Harun*. Edited by Cemâl Kurnâz as *Makâlât-ı Seyyid Hârûn: Tenkitli Basım*. Ankara: Türk Tarih Kurumu Basımevi, 1991.

Abelmann, A. "Cornelis Calkoen op Audiëntie bij Sultan Ahmed III." In *Topkapi en Turkomanie. Turks-Nederlandse Ontmoetingen sinds 1600,* edited by H. Theunissen, A. Abelmann and W. Meulenkamp, pp. 26–36. Amsterdam: Bataafsche Leeuw, 1989.

Abełyan, Manuk. *Hin Kusanakan Žołovrtakan Erger* (Old Popular Minstrel Songs). Yerevan: Armenia S.S.R. Academy of Sciences, 1931.

Abełyan, Manuk, ed. *Sasunc'i Tawit'*. Yerevan: National Press, 1961.

Ådahl, K. "Claes Brorson Rålamb's Embassy to the Sublime Porte in 1657–1658." In *The Sultan's Procession: The Swedish Embassy to Sultan Mehmed IV in 1657–1658 and the Rålamb Paintings,* edited by K. Ådahl, pp. 8–25. Istanbul: Pera Museum, 2006.

Aflaki, Shams al-Din Ahmad. *Manaqib al-'Arifin*. Edited by Tahsin Yazıcı. 2 vols. Ankara: Çaphane-i Encümen-i Tarih-i Türk, 1961.

Ajaryan, H. *Hayeren Armatakan Pararan* (Etymological Dictionary of Armenian). Vol. 4. Yerevan: Yerevan State University, 1979.

Akalin, S. "Kütahya Tiles and Pottery in a Historical Perspective." In *Delights of Kütahya,* pp. 8–15. Istanbul: Suna & Inan Kiraç, 1997.

Allsen, Thomas T. *The Royal Hunt in Eurasian History*. Philadephia: University of Pennsylvania Press, 2006.

Almond, Richard. *Medieval Hunting*. Phoenix Mill: Sutton Publishing Limited, 2003.

Amstrong, P. "The Byzantine and Later Pottery." In *Kalapodi: Ergebnisse der Ausgrabungen im Heiligtum der Artemis und des Apollon von Hyampolis in der antiken Phokis,* edited by R. C. S. Felsch, pp. 336–71. Mainz: Philipp von Zabern, 1996.

And, M. *Istanbul in the 16th Century: The City, The Palace, Daily Life*. Istanbul: Akbank, 1994.

Andrews, Walter G., and Mehmet Kalpaklı. *The Age of Beloveds: Love and the Beloved in Early-Modern Ottoman and European Culture and Society*. Durham, NC: Duke University Press, 2005.

Aqsarayi, Karim al-Din Mahmud b. Muhammad. *Musamirat al-Akhbar va Musa-yirat al-Akhyar*. Edited by Osman Turan. Ankara: Encümen-i Tarih-i Türk, 1943/4.

Araz, N. "Eat Sweet, Talk Sweet." In *Timeless Tastes: Turkish Culinary Culture*, edited by S. Arsel, pp. 19–37. Istanbul: Divan, 1996.

Artan, Tülay. "Art and Architecture." In *The Cambridge History of Turkey*. Vol. 3, *The Later Ottoman Empire, 1603–1839*, edited by Suraiya Faroqhi, pp. 408–80. Cambridge: Cambridge University Press, 2006.

Artan, Tülay. "Aspects of the Ottoman Elite's Food Consumption: Looking for 'Staples,' 'Luxuries,' and 'Delicacies,' in a Changing Century." In *Consumption Studies and the History of the Ottoman Empire, 1550–1922: An Introduction*, edited by Donald Quataert, pp. 107–200. Albany: SUNY Press, 2000.

Artan, Tülay. "Boğaziçi'nin Çehresini Değiştiren Soylu Kadınlar ve Sultanefendi Sarayları." *İstanbul Dergisi* 3 (1992): pp. 109–18.

Artan, Tülay. "A Book of Kings Produced and Presented as a Treatise on Hunting." *Muqarnas* 25 (2008): pp. 299–330.

Asad, Muhammad, trans. and ed. *The Message of the Qur'an*. Gibraltar: Dar al-Andalus, 1997.

Ashiq Pasha, *Gharib-nama*. Edited by Kemal Yavuz as *Garib-nâme: Tıpkıbasım, Karşılaştırmalı Metin ve Aktarma*. İstanbul: Türk Dil Kurumu, 2000.

Ashiq Pashazada, *Tavarikh-i Al-i Osman*. Edited by Çiftçioğlu Nihat Atsız as "Tevârîh-i Âl-i Osman." In *Osmanlı Tarihleri*. İstanbul: Türkiye Yayınevi, 1949, pp. 77–319.

Astarabadi, Aziz b. Ardashir. *Bazm va Razm*. Edited by Fuat Köprülü. İstanbul: Evkaf Matba'ası, 1928.

Atasoy, Nurhan. *1582 Surname-i Hümayun: An Imperial Celebration*. Istanbul: Koçbank, 1997.

Atasoy, Nurhan. *Hasbahçe: Osmanlı Kültüründe Bahçe ve Çiçek*. İstanbul: Koç Kültür Sanat Tanıtım, 2002.

Atasoy, Nurhan, and Julian Raby. *Iznik: The Pottery of Ottoman Turkey*. London: Alexandria Press, 1989.

Atıl, Esin. *Levni and the Surname: The Story of an Eighteenth-Century Ottoman Festival*. Seattle: University of Washington Press, 2000.

Aydın, Halûk. "Ebû Bekr İbnü'l-Hacî Mustafa Kızılhisârî'nin Avcılıkla İlgili bir Eseri: Hidâyetü's Sayyâd." In *Av ve Avcılık Kitabı*, edited by Emine Gürsoy-Naskali and Hilal Oytun Altun, pp. 653–96. İstanbul: Kitabevi Yayınları, 2008.

Ayla, Elif. *Şerbet ve Hoşaf: Hatıralarda Kalan Yudum Yudum Lezzetler*. İstanbul: Hayy Yayınları, 2009.

Azarnoush-Maillard, M. *Islamitisch Aardewerk:* Brussel: Koninklijke Musea voor Kunst en Geschiedenis, 1977.

Baer, Marc D. *Honoured by the Glory of Islam: Conversion and Conquest in Ottoman Europe*. Oxford: Oxford University Press, 2008.

Bağcı, Serpil. "From Translated Word to Translated Image: The Illustrated Şehnâme-i Türkî Copies." *Muqarnas* 17 (2000): pp. 162–76.

Bardakjian, Kevork. *A Reference Guide to Modern Armenian Literature 1500–*

1920. Detroit: Wayne State University Press, 2000.

Bardakjian, Kevork. "The Rise of the Armenian Patriarchate of Constantinople." In *Christians and Jews in the Ottoman Empire,* edited by Benjamin Braude and Bernard Lewis, pp. 89–97. New York: Holmes and Meier, 1982.

Barkan, Ömer Lutfi. "Edirne ve Civarındaki Bazı İmaret Tesislerinin Yıllık Muhasebe Bilançoları." *Belgeler* 1, no. 2 (1964): pp. 235–377.

Barkan, Ömer Lutfi. "Fatih Câmi ve İmareti Tesîslerinin 1489–1490 Yıllarına Âit Muhasebe Bilânçoları." *İstanbul Üniversitesi İktisat Fakültesi Mecmuası* 23, no. 1–2 (1962–63): pp. 297–341.

Barkan, Ömer Lutfi. "İstanbul Saraylarına Ait Muhasebe Defterleri." *Belgeler* IX/13 (1979): pp. 1–370.

Barkan, Ömer Lutfi. "Saray Mutfağının 894–895 (1489–1490) Yılına Âit Muhasebe Bilançosu." *İstanbul Üniversitesi İktisat Fakültesi Mecmuası* 23, no. 1–2 (Ekim–Şubat 1962–63): pp. 380–98.

Barkan, Ömer Lutfi. "Süleymaniye Camii ve İmareti Tesislerine Ait Yıllık bir Muhasebe Bilânçosu 993–994 (1585–1586)." *Vakıflar Dergisi* 9 (1971): pp. 109–62.

Batmanlij, Nacmieh. *From Persia to Napa: Wine at the Persian Table.* Washington DC: Mage Publications, 2006.

Baykal, Kazım. *Bursa ve Anıtları.* Bursa: Aysan Basımevi, 1950.

Beaver, Dan. "The Great Deer Massacre: Animals, Honor, and Communication in Early Modern England." *Journal of British Studies* 38 (1999): pp. 187–216.

Beldiceanu, Nicoară. *Recherche sur la Ville Ottomane au xve Siècle: Étude et Actes.* Paris: A. Maisonneuve, 1953.

Bilgin, Arif. *Osmanlı Tağrasında bir Maliye Kurumu: Bursa Hassa Harç Eminliği.* İstanbul: Kitapevi Yayınları, 2006.

Borromeo, Elisabeth. "The Ottomans and Hunting According to Julien Bordier's Travelogue." In *Animals and People in the Ottoman Empire,* edited by Suraiya Faroqhi, pp. 215–31. Istanbul: Eren Yayınları, 2010.

Brown, D. H. "Class and Rubbish." In *Historical Archaeology: Back from the Edge,* edited by P. P. A. Funari, M. Hall and S. Jones, pp. 151–63. London and New York: Routledge, 1999.

Burckhardt, J. L. *Travels in Nubia.* London: Association for Promoting the Discovery of the Interior Parts of Africa, 1822.

Cantacuzino, Gh. I., and Al. Radulescu. "Betrachtungen über die während dem Jahre 1971 im Kloster Putna geborgene Keramik." *Studii si cercetari de istorie veche* 25 (1974): pp. 527–44.

Caroll, L. "Toward an Archaeology of Non-elite Consumption in Late Ottoman Anatolia." In *A Historical Archaeology of the Ottoman Empire: Breaking New Ground,* edited by U. Baram and L. Caroll, pp. 161–80. New York: Kluwer Academic/Plenum Publishers, 2000.

Caroll, M., D. M. Hadley, and H. Willmott. *Consuming Passions: Dining from An-*

tiquity to the Eighteenth Century. Stroud, Gloucestershire: Tempus, 2005.

Carswell, A. J. "Kütahya Tiles and Ceramics." In *Turkish Tiles and Ceramics*, pp. 50–57. Istanbul: Sadberk Hanim Museum, 1991.

Carswell, A. J. "The Lemon-Squeezer: An Unique Form of Turkish pottery." In *IVème Congrès International d'Art Turc, 1971*, pp. 29–45. Aix-en-Provence: Éditions de l'Université de Provence, 1976.

Carswell, A. J. "Pottery and Tiles on Mount Athos." *Ars Orientalis* 6 (1966): pp. 77–90.

Coşkuner, Fahrettin and Sait Okumuş. "Av ve Avcılığa Dair XV. Yüzyılda Yazılmış bir Av Risalesi: Sayd-name." In *Av ve Avcılık Kitabı,* edited by Emine Gürsoy-Naskali and Hilal Oytun Altun, pp. 697–707. İstanbul: Kitabevi Yayınları, 2008.

Çuhadar, İ. H., ed. *Mustafa Sâfî'nin Zübdetü't-Tevârîh'i*. Vol. 1. Ankara: Türk Tarih Kurumu Yayınları, 2003.

Dadoyan, Seta. "Grigor of Tatev: Treatise against the Tajiks [sic.]." *Islam and Christian-Muslim Relations* 7, no. 2 (1996): pp. 193–204.

de Busbecq, Ogier Ghiselin. *The Turkish Letters of Ogier Ghiselin de Busbecq, Imperial Ambassador at Constantinople 1554–1562*. Translated by Edward Seymour Forster. Baton Rouge: Louisiana State University Press, 2005.

De Groot, A. H. *The Netherlands and Turkey: Four Hundred Years of Political, Economical, Social and Cultural Relations. Selected Essays*. Istanbul: Artpress, 2007.

De Groot, A. H. *The Ottoman Empire and the Dutch Republic: A History of the Earliest Diplomatic Relations 1610–1630*. Leiden: Nederlands Instituut voor het Nabije Oosten, 1978.

Derin, Fahri Ç. *Abdurrahman Abdi Paşa Vekâyî'-Nâmesi (Osmanlı Tarihi [1648–1682])*. İstanbul: Çamlıca Yayınları, 2008.

Dilger, K. *Untersuchungen zur Geschichte des Osmanischen Hoffzeremoniells im 15. und 16. Jahrhundert*. Munich: Rudolph Trofenik, 1967.

Düzdağ, Mehmet Ertuğrul. *Şeyhülislam Ebussud Efendi Fetvaları Işığında 16. Asır Türk Hayatı*. İstanbul: Enderun Kitabevi, 1983.

Ekkart, R. E. O., and Buvelot, Q. *Hollanders in Beeld – Portretten in de Gouden Eeuw*. The Hague: Mauritshuis, 2007.

Elvan Çelebi. *Menâkıbu'l-Kudsiyye fi Menâsıbi'l-Ünsiyye: Baba İlyas-ı Horasânı ve Sülâlesinin Menkabevı Tarihi*. Edited by İsmail Erünsal and Ahmet Yaşar Ocak. Ankara: Türk Tarih Kurumu Basımevi, 1995.

Elvan Çelebi. *Tarihî Metin Çalışmalarında Usul: Menâkıbu'l-Kudsiyye Üzerinde bir Deneme*. Edited by Mertol Tulum. İstanbul: Deniz Kitabevi, 2000.

Enveri. *Le Destan d'Umur Pacha*. Edited and translated to French by Irène Mélikoff. Paris: Presses Universitaires de France, 1954.

Erdbrink, G. R. Bosscha. *At the Threshold of Felicity: Ottoman-Dutch Relations During the Embassy of Cornelis Cakoen at the Sublime Porte 1726–1744*.

Ankara: Türk Tarih Kurumu Basimevi, 1975.

Ergenç, Özer. *XVI. Yüzyılın Sonlarında Bursa: Yerleşimi, Yönetimi, Ekonomik ve Sosyal Durumu Üzerine bir Araştırma.* Ankara: Türk Tarih Kurumu Yayınları, 2006.

Ergenç, Özer. "Osmanlı Klasik Döneminde İstanbul'un Statüsü ve Yönetimi." İstanbul: Paper delivered at the İstanbul'un Fethi ve Fatih Sempozyumu, 14–15 Haziran 2003.

Ergenç, Özer. "The Sphere of *Muqata'a*: A Particular Dimension of Ottoman Spatial Organization and Control." Cambridge: Paper delivered at the İnalcık Conference Harvard University, Spring 2004.

Ergin, Osman N. *Türk Şehirlerinde İmâret Sistemi.* İstanbul: Cumhuriyet Matbaası, 1939.

Ertuğ, Zeynep Tarım. "The Ottoman Imperial Kitchens as Imarets." In *Feeding People, Feeding Power: Imarets in the Ottoman Empire,* edited by Nina Ergin, Christoph K. Neumann, and Amy Singer, pp. 251–59. Istanbul: Eren Yayınları, 2007.

Establet, C., and J. P. Pascual. "Cups, Plates, and Kitchenware in Late Seventeenth- and Early Eighteenth-Century Damascus." In *The Illuminated Table, The Prosperous House: Food and Shelter in Ottoman Material Culture,* edited by Suraiya Faroqhi and Christoph. K. Neumann, pp. 185–197. Würzburg: Ergon Verlag, 2003.

Evliya Çelebi. *Evliya Çelebi Seyahatnamesi.* 10 vols. Edited by Yücel Dağlı, Seyit Ali Kahraman, et al. İstanbul: Yapı Kredi Yayınları, 1996–2007.

Evliya Çelebi. *Narrative of Travels in Europe, Asia and Africa in the Seventeenth Century.* Translated by Joseph von Hammer. 2 vols. London: Printed for the Oriental Translation Fund of Great Britain and Ireland, 1846–50.

Fahriye, Ayşe. *Ev Kadını.* Translated by Leman Erdemli and Zeynep Vanlı. İstanbul: Ofset Yapımevi, 2002. Originally published by Dersaadet: Arif Efendi Matbaası, 1323 [1905/6].

Faroqhi, Suraiya. "Agricultural Crisis and the Art of Flute-Playing: The Worldly Affairs of the Mevlevî Dervishes (1595–1652)." *Turcica* 20 (1988): pp. 43–70.

Faroqhi, Suraiya. "Introduction." In *The Illuminated Table, the Prosperous House: Food and Shelter in Ottoman Material Culture,* edited by Suraiya Faroqhi and Christoph K. Neumann, pp. 9–33. Wüzburg: Ergon-Verlag, 2003.

Faroqhi, Suraiya. *Subjects of the Sultan: Culture and Daily Life in the Ottoman Empire.* London: I.B. Tauris, 2000.

Finkel, C. *Osman's Dream. The Story of the Ottoman Empire 1300–1923.* London: John Murray, 2005.

Fletcher, Nicola. *Charlemagne's Tablecloth. A Piquant History of Feasting.* New York: Saint Martin's Press, 2005.

Frantz, M. A. "Turkish Pottery from the Agora." *Hesperia* 11 (1942): pp. 1–28.

Freifrau von Müffling, Sonja. "Cooking with Game." In *Game and Hunting*, edited by Kurt G. Blüchel, pp. 586–613. Cologne: Könemann, 1977.

Friedlander, Shams. *The Whirling Dervishes*. Albany: SUNY Press, 1992.

Froom, Aimée E. "Adorned Like a Rose: The Persian Connection in the *Muraqqa* for the Ottoman Sultan Murad III (Austrian National Library, Cod. Mixt. 313)." *Artibus Asiae* 66/2 (2006): pp. 137–54.

Froom, Aimée E. "Collecting Tastes: A Muraqqa' for Sultan Murad III." *Electronic Journal of Oriental Studies* IV (2001).

Gerlach, S. *Stephan Gerlachs dess Aeltern Tage-buch. . .* Frankfurt am Main: Johann-David Zunners, 1674.

Gerö, G. "Türkische Keramik in Ungarn, Einheimische und Importierten Waren." In *Fifth International Congress of Turkish Art*, edited by G. Feher, pp. 363–84. Budapest: Akademiai Kiado, 1978.

Ghougassian, Vazken S. *The Emergence of the Armenian Diocese of New Julfa in the Seventeenth Century*. Atlanta: Scholars Press, 1998.

Gölpınarlı, Abdülbâki. *Mevlânâ'dan sonra Mevlevîlik*. İstanbul: İnkılâp Kitabevi, 1983.

Goody, J. *Cooking, Cuisine and Class. A Study in Comparative Sociology*. Cambridge: Cambridge University Press, 1982.

Gülşehri. *Gülschehrîs Mesnevi auf Achi Evran, den Heiligen von Kirschehir und Patron der türkischen Zünfte*. Edited by Franz Taeschner. Wiesbaden: Franz Steiner Verlag, 1955.

Hacı Bektâş Veli. *Vilâyet-nâme: Manâkıb-ı Hünkâr Hacı Bektâş-ı Veli*. Edited by Abdülbâkî Gölpınarlı with a MS. facsimile. 2nd ed. İstanbul: İnkılâp, 1995.

Hacikyan, Agop J., et al., eds. *The Heritage of Armenian Literature*. Detroit: Wayne State University Press, 2005.

Halıcı, Feyzi. *Ali Eşref Dede'nin Yemek Risalesi*. Ankara: Atatürk Kültür Merkezi Yayınları, 1992.

Hayes, J. W. *Excavations at Saraçhane in Istanbul*. Vol. 2, *The Pottery*. Washington, D.C.: Dumbarton Oaks, 1992.

Heal, Felicity. "Food Gifts, the Household and the Politics of Exchange in Early Modern England." *Past and Present* 199 (May 2008): pp. 41–70.

Heyd, Uriel. *Ottoman Documents on Palestine 1552–1615*. Oxford: Oxford University Press, 1960.

Hoenkamp-Mazgon, M. *Palais de Hollande in Istanbul: The Embassy and Envoys of The Netherlands since 1612*. Amsterdam and Istanbul: Boom, 2001.

Huggins, P. J. "Excavations at Sewardstone Street, Walthan Abbey, Essex 1966." *Post-Medieval Archaeology* 3 (1969): pp. 47–99.

Ibn Batuta. *Voyages d'Ibn Batoutah*. Edited and translated by C. Defrémery and B. R. Sanguinetti. 4vols. Paris: Société Asiatique, 1877.

Ibn Fadl Allah al-'Umari, Ahmad b. Yahya. *Masalik al-Absar fi Mamalik al-Amsar*. Edited by Ahmad 'Abd al-Qadir al-Shadhali. Abu Dhabi: al-Majma' al-Thafaqi, 2003.

İnalcık, Halil. "Bursa XV. Asır Sanayi ve Ticaret Tarihine Dair Vesikalar." *Belleten* 24 (1960): pp. 45–102.

İnalcık, Halil. "Capital Formation in the Ottoman Empire." *Journal of Economic History* 29/1 (1969): pp. 97–140.

İrepoğlu, G. *Levni. Painting, Poetry, Colour.* Istanbul: Republic of Turkey Ministry of Culture, 1999.

Işın, E. "Coffeehouses as Places of Conversation." In *The Illuminated Table, The Prosperous House: Food and Shelter in Ottoman Material Culture*, edited by Suraiya Faroqhi and Christoph K. Neumann, pp. 199–208. Würzburg: Ergon Verlag, 2003.

Kafadar, C. "The City That Rålamb Visited: The Political and Cultural Climate of Istanbul in the 1650s." In *The Sultan's Procession: The Swedish Embassy to Sultan Mehmed IV in 1657–1658 and the Rålamb Paintings*, edited by K. Ådahl, pp. 59–73. Istanbul: Pera Museum, 2006.

Karamustafa, Ahmet. *God's Unruly Friends: Dervish Groups in the Islamic Later Middle Period, 1200–1550.* Salt Lake City: University of Utah Press, 1994.

Kaykavus b. Iskandar b. Qabus. *The Book of Advice by King Kay Kâ'us ibn Iskander: The Earliest Old Ottoman Turkish version of his Qâbûsnâme.* Edited by Eleazar Birnbaum. Sources of Oriental Languages and Literatures 6. Duxbury, MA: Şinasi Tekin and Gönül Alpay Tekin, 1981.

Keskin, Yusuf Ziya. "Hadislere Göre Avlanma Kuralları." In *Av ve Avcılık Kitabı*, edited by Emine Gürsoy-Naskali and Hilal Oytun Altun, pp. 497–514. İstanbul: Kitabevi Yayınları, 2008.

Khane, Meera. "The Wine-Cup in Mughal Court Culture: From Hedonism to Kingship." *The Medieval History Journal* 8 (2005): pp. 143–88.

Kiel, M. "Byzantine Architecture and Painting in Central Greece 1460–1570." *Byzantinische Forschungen* 16 (1990): pp. 429–46.

Kindermann, H., ed., *Uber die guten Sitten beim Essen und Trinken: Das ist das Buch von Al-Ghazzali's Hauptwerk.* Leiden: Brill, 1964.

Klein, Yaron. "Between Public and Private: An Examination of *Hisba* Literature." *Harvard Middle Eastern and Islamic Review* 7 (2006): pp. 41–62.

Koch, Ebba. *Dara-Shikoh Shooting Nilgais: Hunt and Landscape in Mughal Painting.* Occasional Papers. Washington: Freer Gallery of Art, 1998.

Kolodziejczyk, D. "Polish Embassies in Istanbul, or: How to Sponge on Your Host Without Losing Your Self-esteem." In *The Illuminated Table, The Prosperous House: Food and Shelter in Ottoman Material Culture*, edited by Suraiya Faroqhi and Christoph K. Neumann, pp. 51–58. Würzburg: Ergon Verlag, 2003.

Korre-Zographou, K. *Ta Kerameika Tou Ellinikou Chorou.* Athens: Ekdotikos Oikos Melissa, 1995.

Kourkoutidou, E., Chr. Tsioumi, and Th. Pazaras. "Excavations at Thessaloniki" (in Modern Greek). *Archaiologikon Deltion* 31 (1976 = 1984): pp. 267–70, pls. 210–13.

Krahl, R., N. Erbahar, and J. Ayers. *Chinese Ceramics in the Topkapı Saray Museum, Istanbul: A Complete Catalogue.* New York: Sotheby's Publications, 1986.

Kuran, Abdullah. "A Spatial Study of Three Ottoman Capitals: Bursa, Edirne, and Istanbul." *Muqarnas* 13 (1996): pp. 114–31.

Kürkçüoğlu, Kemal Edib. *Süleymaniye Vakfiyesi.* Ankara: Resimli Posta Matbaası, 1962.

Kuru, Selim S. "Naming the Beloved in Ottoman Turkish Gazel: The Case of İshak Çelebi (d. 1537/8)." In *Ghazal as World Literature.* Vol. 2, II. *From a Literary Genre to a Great Tradition: The Ottoman Gazel in Context,* edited by Angelika Neuwirth, Michael Hess, Judith Pfeiffer, and Boerte Sagaster, pp. 163–173. Beirut: Ergon Verlag, 2005–2006.

Kuru, Selim S. "Sex in the Text: Deli Birader's Dâfi'ü'l-Gumûm ve Râfi'ü 'l-Humûm and the Ottoman Literary Canon." *Middle Eastern Literatures* 10/2 (2007): pp. 157–74.

Kut, G. "Turkish Culinary Culture." In *Timeless Tastes. Turkish Culinary Culture,* edited by S. Arsel, pp. 38–61. Istanbul: Divan, 1996.

Kütükoğlu, Mübahat. *Osmanlılarda Narh Müessesesi ve 1640 Tarihli Narh Defteri.* Istanbul: Enderun Kitabevi, 1983.

Laine, M. "Audienstavlorna på Biby." In *Minnet av Konstantinopel. Den Osmansk-Turkiska 1700-Tallssamlingen på Biby,* edited by K. Ådahl et al., pp. 113–45. Stockholm: Atlantis, 2003.

Lane, A. *Later Islamic Pottery: Persia, Syria, Egypt, Turkey.* 2nd ed. London: Faber & Faber, 1971.

Lane, A. "Turkish Peasant Pottery from Chanak and Kutahia." *The Connoisseur* 104 (1939): pp. 232–59.

Laufer, Berthold. "On the Possible Oriental Origin of Our Word Booze." *Journal of the American Oriental Society* 49 (1929): pp. 56–58.

Lewis, Franklin. *Rumi Past and Present, East and West: The Life, Teachings and Poetry of Jalâl al-Din Rumi.* Oxford: Oneworld, 2000.

Lowry, Heath. *Ottoman Bursa in Travel Accounts.* Bloomington: Indiana University Ottoman and Modern Turkish Studies Publications, 2003.

Luttervelt, R. Van. *De 'Turkse' Schilderijen van J.B. Vanmour en zijn School: De Verzameling van Cornelis Calkoen, Ambassadeur bij de Hoge Porte, 1725–1743.* Istanbul: Nederlands Historisch Archeologisch Instituut in het Nabije Oosten, 1958.

Madoyan, A., and G. Ananian, eds. *Hayoc' hin ew Mijnadarean Banastelcut'ean Krestomatia* (Anthology of Ancient and Medieval Armenian Poetry). Yerevan: Yerevan State University, 1979.

Malxaseanc', S. *Hayeren Bac'atrakan Baṙaran* (Armenian Descriptive Dictionary). Vol. 4. Yerevan: Armenian National Press, 1945.

Manning, Roger B. *Hunters and Poachers: A Social and Cultural History of Un-*

lawful Hunting in England, 1485–1640. Oxford: Oxford University Press, 1993.

Mansel, Ph. *Constantinople: City of the World's Desire 1453–1924*. London: John Murray, 1995.

Manukyan, A. S., ed. *Hayeren Jeṙagreri hišatakaranner JG daṙ*. Yerevan: Armenian Academy of Sciences, 1984.

Margos, A. "Die Armenische Kirche Heiliger Stephanos in der Stadt Provadya." *Bulletin du Musée National de Varna* 12 (1976): pp. 137–39.

Megaw, A. H. S. "Three Medieval Pit-groups from Nicosia." *Report of Antiquities, Cyprus 1937–39* (1937 = 1951): pp. 145–68 and 224–26.

Meier, Astrid. "For the Sake of God Alone? Food Distribution Policies, *Takiyya*s and Imarets in Early Ottoman Damascus." In *Feeding People, Feeding Power: Imarets in the Ottoman Empire*, edited by Nina Ergin, Christoph K. Neumann, and Amy Singer, pp. 121–50. Istanbul: Eren Yayınları, 2007.

Mennel, S. *All Manners of Food: Eating and Taste in England and France from the Middle Ages to the Present*. Oxford: Basil Blackwell, 1985.

Meredith-Owens, G. M. *Turkish Miniatures*. London: British Museum Publications, 1963.

Milstein, Rachel. *Miniature Painting in Ottoman Baghdad*. Costa Mesa: Mazda Publications, 1990.

Misugi, T. *Chinese Porcelain Collections in the Near East: Topkapı and Ardebil*. Vol. 1. Hong Kong: Hong Kong University Press, 1981.

Mnac'akanyan, Asatur. *Hayrenner* (Hayrens). Yerevan: Matenadaran, 1995.

Montagu, Mary Wortley. *The Complete Letters of Lady Mary Wortley Montagu*. Edited by Robert Halsband. 3 vols. Oxford: Clarendon Press, 1966–67.

Muhammad Ibn Al-Hasan Ibn Muhammad Ibn Al-Karîm. *A Baghdad Cookery Book: The Book of Dishes (Kitâb al-Tabîkh)*. Translated by Charles Perry. Trowbridge, UK: Cromwell Press, 2005.

Muhammad Ibn al-Ukhuwwa. *Ma'alim al-Qurba fi Ahkamm al-Hisba*. Edited by Muhammad Mahmud Sha'ban et al. Cairo: al-Hai'a al-Misriya, 1976.

Muhammed bin Mahmud Şirvani. 15. Yüzyıl Osmanlı Mutfağı. Edited by Mustafa Argunşah and Müjgan Çakır. İstanbul: Gökkubbe Yayınları, 2005.

Mustafa, Celalzâde. "Tabaqât ül-Memâlik ve Derecât ül-Mesâlik." In *Geschichte Sultan Süleyman Kanunis von 1520 bis 1557*, edited by Petra Kappert. Wiesbaden: Franz Steiner Verlag, 1981.

Mustafa Ali. *Mustafā Ālī's Counsel for Sultans of 1581*. Edited and translated by Andreas Tietze. Vol. 2. Vienna: Verlag der Österreichischen Akademie der Wissenschaften, 1982.

Mustafa Ali. *The Ottoman Gentleman of the Sixteenth Century: Mustafa Âli's Mevâ'idü'n-Nefâ'is fî Kavâ'idi'l-Mecâlis: "Tables of Delicacies Concerning the Rules of Social Gatherings."* Annotated English Translation by Douglas S. Brookes. Sources of Oriental Languages and Literatures 59. Cambridge,

MA: Department of Near Eastern Languages and Civilizations, 2003.

Necipoğlu, G. *Architecture, Ceremonial, and Power: The Topkapı Palace in the Fifteenth and Sixteenth Centuries.* Cambridge, MA, and London: The Architectural History Foundation, 1991.

Nikolakopoulos, G. A. "The Ceramics of the Chapel of Phaneromeni of Salamis." *Archaiologia* 28 (1988): pp. 81–84.

Nikolakopoulos, G. A. "Embedded Ceramics of Churches." *Archaiologia* 33 (1989): pp. 66–71.

Öcalan, Hasan Basri. "Bursa'da Boza ve Tarihi Bozahaneler." In *I. Bursa Halk Kültürü Sempozyumu Bildiri Kitabi,* edited by Y. Oğuzoğlu and K. Üstünova, vol. 1, 111–22. Bursa: Bursa University Press, 2002.

Pancaroğlu, Oya. "Architecture, Landcape, and Patronage in Bursa: The Making of an Ottoman Capital City." *Turkish Studies Association Bulletin* 20, no. 1 (1995): pp. 40–55.

Piscowicz, Andrzej. "How Did New Persian and Arabic Words Penetrate the Middle Armenian Vocabulary? Remarks on the Material of Kostandin Erznkaci'is Poetry." In *New Approaches to Medieval Armenian Language and Literature,* edited by J. J. S. Weitenberg, pp. 95–110. Amsterdam: Rodopi B.V., 1995.

Pitari-Mayioletti, E. "Some European-made Treasures of Skyros." *Zygos* 4 (1973): pp. 6–9.

Ravendî, Muhammed b. Ali b. Süleyman, er-. *Râhat-üs-Sudûr ve Âyet-üs-Sürûr.* Vol. 2. Translated by Ahmet Ateş. Ankara: Türk Tarih Kurumu, 1960.

Raye, J. *Een Levenslustig Heer op Reis Naar de Oriënt: Brieven van Johan Raye, Heer van Breukelerwaart 1764–1769.* Baarn: Bosch&Keuning, 1987.

Reindl-Kiel, H. "The Chickens of Paradise: Official Meals in the Mid-Seventeenth-Century Ottoman Palace." In *The Illuminated Table, The Prosperous House: Food and Shelter in Ottoman Material Culture,* edited by Suraiya Faroqhi and Christoph K. Neumann, pp. 59–88. Würzburg: Ergon Verlag, 2003.

Reindl-Kiel, H. "Die Lippen der Geliebten: Betrachtungen zur Geschichte der türkischen Küche." *Mitteilungen der Deutsch-Türkische Gesellschaft* 116 (1993): pp. 13–23.

Rogers, M. "Archaeology vs. Archives: Some Recent Approaches to the Ottoman Pottery of Iznik." In *The Balance of Truth: Essays in Honour of Professor Geoffrey Lewis,* edited by Ç. Balım-Harding and C. Imber, pp. 275–92. Istanbul: Isis Press, 2000.

Rogers, M. "Plate and its Substitutes in Ottoman Inventories." In *Pots & Pans: A Colloquium on Precious Metals and Ceramics in the Muslim, Chinese and Graeco-Roman Worlds,* edited by M. Vickers, pp. 117–36. Oxford: Oxford University Press, 1986.

Rossant, Julliette. "The World's First Soft Drink." *Saudi Aramco World* 56/5 (September–October 2005): pp. 36–39.

Russell, James. "The Praise of Porridge." In *Le Muséon,* 116, nos. 1–2 (2003): pp. 137–79.

Russell, James R. *Yovhannēs Tłkuranc 'i and the Mediaeval Armenian Lyric Tradition.* Atlanta: Scholars Press, 1987.

Sahakyan, H., ed. *Uš Miĵnadari hay Banastełcut 'yunə (XVI–XVII dd.).* Vol. 2. Yerevan: Armenia S.S.R. Academy of Sciences, 1987.

Samancı, Ö. "Culinary Consumption Patterns of the Ottoman Elite During the First Half of the Nineteenth Century." In *The Illuminated Table, The Prosperous House: Food and Shelter in Ottoman Material Culture,* edited by Suraiya Faroqhi and Christopher K. Neumann, pp. 161–84. Würzburg: Ergon Verlag, 2003.

Samancı, Ö. "19. Yüzyıl Istanbul Mutfağı'nda Yeni Lezzetler." *Yemek ve Kültür* 6 (2006): pp. 86–96.

Sancisi-Weerdenburg, H. "De Oorsprong van een 'Haute Cuisine'." *Phoenix* 43, no. 2 (1997): pp. 93–102.

Sanjian, Avedis K., ed. *Colophons of Armenian Manuscripts* (Cambridge, MA: Harvard University Press, 1969.

Savkay, T. "The Cultural and Historic Context of Turkish Cuisine." In *Timeless Tastes: Turkish Culinary Culture,* edited by S. Arsel, pp. 75–88. Istanbul: Divan, 1996.

Scarce, J. *Domestic Culture in the Middle East: An Exploration of the Household Interior.* Edinburgh: National Museums of Scotland, 1996.

Schiendlein, Raymond. "Hebrew Poetry in Medieval Iberia." In *Convivencia: Jews, Muslims and Christians in Medieval Spain,* edited by Vivian B. Mann et al., pp. 39–60. New York: George Braziller in association with the Jewish Museum, 1992.

Schweigger, Salomon. *Sultanlar Kentine Yolculuk 1578–1581.* İstanbul: Kitap Yayınevi, 2004.

Sefercioğlu, M. Nejat. *Türk Yemekleri: XVIII. Yüzyıla Ait bir Yemek Risâlesi.* Ankara: Kültür ve Turizm Bakanlığı, 1985.

Şen, Mesut. "Geyik." In *Av ve Avcılık Kitabı,* edited by Emine Gürsoy-Naskali and Hilal Oytun Altun, pp. 75–88. İstanbul: Kitabevi Yayınları, 2008.

Şentürk, Ahmet Atilla. "Osmanlı Şiirinde Aşka Dair." *Doğu Batı* 7/26 (2004): pp. 55–68

Sertoğlu, Midhat. *Osmanlı Tarih Luğatı.* İstanbul: Enderun Kitabevi, 1986.

Shepherd, Dorothy G. "Banquet and Hunt in Medieval Islamic Iconography." In *Gatherings in Honor of Dorothy E. Miner,* edited by Ursula E. McCracken, Lilian M.C. Randall, and Richard H. Randall, Jr., pp. 79–94. Baltimore: The Walters Art Gallery, 1974.

Sılay, Kemal. "Ahmedî's History of the Ottoman Dynasty." *Journal of Turkish Studies* 16 (1992): pp. 129–200.

Sılay, Kemal. *Nedim and the Poetics of the Ottoman Court: Medieval Inheritance and the Need for Change.* Bloomington: Indiana University, 1994.

Singer, Amy. *Charity in Islamic Societies.* Cambridge: Cambridge University Press, 2008.

Singer, Amy. *Constructing Ottoman Beneficence: An Imperial Soup Kitchen in Jerusalem*. Albany: State University of New York Press, 2002.

Singer, Amy. "Imarets." In *The Ottoman World*, edited by Christine Woodhead. London: Routledge, forthcoming.

Sint Nicolaas, Eveline. "The Ambassador and the Sultan." In *The Ambassador, the Sultan and the Artist: An Audience in Istanbul*, pp. 3–17. Amsterdam and Zwolle: Rijksmuseum & Waanders, 2003.

Sint Nicolaas, Eveline, Duncan Bull, and Günsel Renda. *The Ambassador, the Sultan and the Artist: An Audience in Istanbul*. Amsterdam and Zwolle: Rijksmuseum & Waanders, 2003.

Sint Nicolaas, Eveline, Duncan Bull, Günsel Renda, and Gül İrepoğlu. *An Eyewitness of the Tulip Era: Jean-Baptiste Vanmour*. Istanbul: Koçbank, 2003.

Sipahsalar, Faridun b. Ahmad. *Risala-yi Faridun b. Ahmad Sipahsalar dar Ahval-i Mavlana Jalal al-Din Mavlavi*. Edited by Sa'id Nafisi. Tehran: Kitabkhana va Chapkhana-yi Iqbal, 1320 [1941–2].

Şirvani, Muhammed bin Mahmud. *15. Yüzyıl Osmanlı Mutfağı: Muhammed bin Mahmûd Şirvanî*. Edited by Mustafa Argunşah and Müjgan Çakır. İstanbul: Gökkubbe Yayınları, 2005.

Slot, J. "De diplomatieke betrekkingen tussen Nederland en het Osmaanse Rijk." In *Topkapı en Turkomanie: Turks-Nederlandse Ontmoetingen sinds 1600*, edited by H. Theunissen, A. Abelmann and W. Meulenkamp, pp. 9–25. Amsterdam: Bataafsche Leeuw, 1989.

Sparapet, Smpat. *Datastanagirk'* (Law Code). Edited by A. Galstyan. Yerevan: Armenia S.S.R. Academy of Sciences, Yerevan, 1958.

Spence, Jonathan D. *Emperor of China: Self-Portrait of K'ang-his*. New York: Vintage Books, 1974.

Stephan, St. H. "An Endowment Deed of Khâsseki Sultân, Dated 24th May 1552." *Quarterly of the Department of Antiquities in Palestine* 10 (1944): pp. 170–94.

Surmelian, Leon, transl. *Daredevils of Sassoun*. Denver: Alan Swallow, 1964.

Syson, Luke, and Dillian Gordon. *Pisanello: Painter to the Renaissance Court*. London: National Gallery Co Ltd, 2002.

Tabîb İbn-i Şerîf. *15. Yüzyıl Türkçe Tıb Kitabı: Yadigâr-ı İbn-i Şerîf*. Edited by M. Yahya Okutan, Doğan Koçer, and Mecit Yıldız. İstanbul: Yerküre Yayınları, 2004.

Tat'ewac'i, Grigor. *Girk' Harc'manc'* (Book of Questions). Constantinople: [Astowacatowr Kostandnowpolsec'i], 1729.

Tezcan, Semih. *Bir Ziyafet Defteri*. İstanbul: Simurg Yayınları, 1998.

Thiel, P. J. J. van. *Alle Schilderijen van het Rijksmuseum te Amsterdam: Volledig Geïllustreerde Catalogus*, pp. 741–50. Amsterdam and Haarlem: Rijksmuseum, 1976.

Thomson, Robert. "Muhammad and the Origin of Islam in the Armenian Literary

Tradition." In *Armenian Studies in Memoriam Haig Berberian,* edited by Kouymjian, Dickran, 829–58. Lisbon: Calouste Gulbenkian Foundation, 1986.

Thomson, Robert, ed. *The Lawcode [Datastanagirk'] of Mxit'ar Goš.* Atlanta: Editions Rodopi, 2000.

Ünver, A. Süheyl. *Fatih Devri Yemekleri.* İstanbul: İstanbul Üniversitesi Tıp Tarihi Enstitüsü, 1952.

Ursinus, M. "Die Ess- und Trinkgewohnheiten der Osmanen." In *Türkische Kunst und Kultur aus Osmanischer Zeit,* pp. 155–58. Recklinghausen: Museum für Kunsthandwerk der Stadt Frankfurt, 1985.

Uvezian, Sona. *The Cuisine of Armenia.* New York: Hippocrene Books, 1974.

Vavylopoulou-Charitonidou, A. "Céramique d'Offrande Trouvée dans des Tombes Byzantines Tardives de l'Hippodrome de Thessalonique." In *Recherches sur la Céramique Byzantine. Bulletin du Correspondance Hellénique* Suppl. 18, edited by V. Déroche and J. M. Spieser, pp. 209–25. Athens: École Française d'Athènes, 1989.

Viré, François. "Jurisprudence en Matière de Gibier Tué à Plomb: *Risâla Tuhfat al-Hawass fî Hill Sayd Bunduq al-Rasâs." Bulletin d'études orientales* 30 (1978): pp. 289–305.

Vroom, J. *After Antiquity: Ceramics and Society in the Aegean from Circa the 7th to the 20th centuries A. C.: A Case Study from Boeotia, Central Greece.* Archaeological Studies Leiden University 10. Leiden: Leiden University, 2003.

Vroom, J. "Breaking Pots: Medieval and Post-Medieval Ceramics from Central Greece." In *Medieval and Post-Medieval Greece: The Corfu Papers,* edited by J. Bintliff and H. Stöger, pp. 167–76. Oxford: Oxbow Books, 2009.

Vroom J. "Byzantine Garbage and Ottoman Waste." In *Thèbes: Fouilles de la Cadmée. II.2. Les Tablettes en Linéaire B de la 'Odos Pelopidou': La Céramique de la Odos Pelopidou et la Chronologie du Linéaire B,* edited by E. Andrikou, V. L. Aravantinos, L. Godard, A. Sacconi, and J. Vroom, pp. 181–233. Pisa and Rome: Instituti Editoriali e Poligrafici Internazionali, 2006.

Vroom J. "Byzantine Garlic and Turkish Delight: Dining Habits and Cultural Change in Central Greece from Byzantine to Ottoman Times." *Archaeological Dialogues* 7 (2000): pp. 199–216.

Vroom, J. *Byzantine to Modern Pottery in the Aegean: An Introduction and Field Guide.* Utrecht: Parnassus Press, 2005.

Vroom J. "Coffee and Archaeology: A Note on a Kütahya Ware Find in Boeotia, Greece." *Pharos (Journal of the Netherlands Institute at Athens)* 4 (1996): pp. 5–19.

Vroom J. "Kütahya Between the Lines: Post-Medieval Ceramics as Historical Information." In *Between Venice and Istanbul: Colonial Landscapes in Early Modern Greece,* edited by S. Davies and J. Davis, pp. 71–93. Hesperia Supplement 40. Princeton: The American School of Classical Studies at Athens, 2007.

Vroom, J. "Medieval and Post-Medieval Pottery from a Site in Boeotia: A Case Study Example of Post-Classical Archaeology in Greece." *Annual of the British School at Athens* 93 (1998): pp. 513–46.

Waagé, F. O. "The Roman and Byzantine Pottery." *Hesperia* 2 (1933): pp. 279–328.

Waines, D., H. İnalcik, and J. Burton-Page. "Maṭbakh." In *Encyclopaedia of Islam*, 2nd ed., 6:809–13. Leiden: Brill, 1960–2003.

Wartburg. M. L. von, "Types of Imported Tableware at Kouklia in the Ottoman Period." *Report of the Department of Antiquities, Cyprus* (2001): pp. 361–396.

Watson, O. "Ceramics." In *Islamic Art in the Keir Collection*, edited by B. W. Robinson, pp. 137–286. London: Faber Ltd., 1980.

Wellesz, Emmy. "Die Miniaturen im Album Murad III." *Wiener Beitrage Zur Kunst und Kulturgeschichte Asiens 10* (1936): pp. 55–67.

Westerberg, S. "Claes Rålamb: Statesman, Scholar and Ambassador." In *The Sultan's Procession: The Swedish Embassy to Sultan Mehmed IV in 1657–1658 and the Rålamb Paintings*, edited by K. Ådahl, pp. 26–57. Istanbul: Pera Museum, 2006.

Woolgar, Chris. "Diet and Consumption in Gentry and Noble Households: A Case Study From Around the Wash." In *Rulers and Ruled in Late Medieval England: Essays Presented to Gerald Harris*, edited by Rowena E. Archer and Simon Walker, pp. 17–32. London: Hambledon Press, 1995.

Yarshater, Ehsan. "The Theme of Wine-Drinking and the Concept of the Beloved in Early Persian Poetry." *Studia Islamica* 13 (1960): pp. 43–53.

Yerasimos, Stephanos. *Sultan Sofraları: 15. ve 16. Yüzyılda Osmanlı Saray Mutfağı*. İstanbul: Yapı ve Kredi Yayınları, 2002.

Yi, Eunjeong. *Guild Dynamics in Seventeenth-Century Istanbul: Fluidity and Leverage*. Leiden and Boston: Brill, 2004.

Yılmaz, Fikret. "Boş Vaktınız Var Mı? Veya 16. Yüzyılda Anadolu'da Şarap, Eğlence ve Suç." *Tarih ve Toplum: Yeni Yaklaşımlar* 1/241 (2005): pp. 11–49.

Yılmazer, Ziya, ed. *Topçular Kâtibi 'Abdülkâdir (Kadri) Efendi Tarihi*. Ankara: Türk Tarih Kurumu Yayınları, 2003.

Index

About the Editor and Contributors

Nicolas Trépanier is an assistant professor in the Department of History at the University of Mississippi. He completed his dissertation, "Food as a Window into Daily Life in Fourteenth Century Central Anatolia," at Harvard University (2008).

İklil O. Selçuk completed her dissertation, "State and Society in the Marketplace: A Study of Late Fifteenth-Century Bursa," at Harvard University (2009). She teaches European and Ottoman Economic History in the Department of Economics at Bahçeşehir University in Istanbul.

Rachel Goshgarian is Director of the Krikor and Clara Zohrab Information Center of the Diocese of the Armenian Church of America (Eastern). She completed her dissertation, "Beyond the Social and the Spiritual: Redefining the Urban Confraternities of Late Medieval Anatolia," at Harvard University (2008).

Amy Singer is a professor in the Department of Middle Eastern and African History at Tel Aviv University. She is the author of *Palestinian Peasants and Ottoman Officials: Rural Administration around Sixteenth-Century Jerusalem* (1994), *Constructing Ottoman Beneficence: An Imperial Soup Kitchen in Jerusalem* (2002), and *Charity in Islamic Societies* (2008).

Tülay Artan is on the Faculty of Arts and Social Sciences, Sabancı University. Her publications include "A Book of Kings Produced and Presented as a Treatise on Hunting," *Muqarnas: An Annual on the Visual Culture of the Islamic World* 25 (December 2008), and "Arts and Architecture," *The Cambridge History of Turkey*, vol. 3, *The Later Ottoman Empire, 1603–1839* (2006).

Joanita A. C. Vroom, Ph.D., is the VIDI Research Project Leader at the Amsterdam Archaeological Centre in the Faculty of Humanities at the University of Amsterdam. She is the author of *After Antiquity: Ceramics and Society in the Aegean from the 7th to 20th Century A.C., A Case Study from Boeotia, Central Greece* (2003) and *Byzantine to Modern Pottery in the Aegean: 7th to 20th Century: An Introduction and Field Guide* (2006).

573

LaVergne, TN USA
03 November 2010
203377LV00002B/4/P

9 781558 765146